D0189426

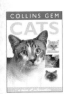

COLLINS GEM
CATS
a mine of information

COLLINS GEM
Chinese
ASTROLOGY
牛 虎 兔
a mine of information

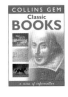

COLLINS GEM
Classic
BOOKS
a mine of information

COLLINS GEM
Classic
FILMS
a mine of information

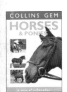

COLLINS GEM
HORSES
& PONIES
a mine of information

COLLINS GEM
INSECTS
a mine of information

COLLINS GEM
KINGS &
QUEENS
a mine of information

COLLINS GEM
MUSHROOMS
& TOADSTOOLS
a mine of information

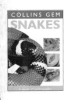

COLLINS GEM
SNAKES
a mine of information

COLLINS GEM
SPIDERS
a mine of information

COLLINS GEM
STRESS
Survival Guide
a mine of information

COLLINS GEM
TAROT
a mine of information

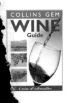

COLLINS GEM
WINE
Guide
a mine of information

COLLINS GEM
WORLD
atlas
a mine of information

COLLINS GEM
YOGA
a mine of information

COLLINS GEM
ZODIAC
Types
a mine of information

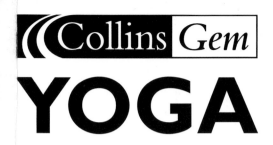

Collins Gem

YOGA

Patricia A. Ralston
Caroline Smart

HarperCollins*Publishers*

Patricia A. Ralston is a qualified hatha yoga teacher with
10 years' experience of teaching. She is also a holistic
therapist, practising the therapies of reflexology, aromatherapy
and massage.
Caroline Smart has been practising yoga for over 20 years.

Posture illustrations by Fiona C. Steel
Other illustrations by David Braysher

HarperCollins Publishers
Westerhill Road, Bishopbriggs,Glasgow G64 2QT

First published 1999

Reprint 10 9 8 7 6 5 4

© The Printer's Devil (text and illustrations) 1999

ISBN 0 00 472320-1

Printed in Italy by Amadeus S.p.A.

Introduction

Many people are wary of yoga, either imagining it as a type of weird Eastern religion or else seeing it as a form of soft physical exercise practised by middle-aged ladies. Consequently, yoga is sometimes ridiculed or dismissed out of hand. But once discovered for what it is – an extremely effective and beneficial form of exercise, both for the body and mind – the student will incorporate yoga almost unconsciously into his or her way of life.

Yoga brings not only an awareness to your body – how you sit, how you stand, how you breathe – but it also focuses your attention on your mind, letting you learn how to relax.

If you can, try to approach yoga without any preconceptions. You can take from it as much or as little as you want. If you just want something to make you more supple then attend a beginner's class and feel the gentle stretching you can get from practising the postures. You may find yourself wanting to explore other aspects of yoga: the breathing, the philosophy, the literature. As much or as little as you want is there to be discovered. But just as your yoga teacher will tell you when referring to the postures, 'Only do what feels right for you'.

The selection of postures included in this book have been chosen to illustrate the ones that are likely to be taught in a hatha yoga class. We have omitted some of the more difficult postures which should be learned under the supervision of a qualified yoga teacher.

HATHA YOGA

> *Asanas are spoken of first, being the first stage of
> hatha yoga. So one should practise the asanas which
> give strength, keep him in good health, and make
> his limbs supple.*
> Hatha Yoga Pradipika

What is Hatha Yoga?

This chapter is an introduction to hatha yoga, the type
you will probably be practising; More About Yoga (*p.
182*) details the range of types of yoga and practice.

In the West, yoga usually means hatha yoga. This is
the physical side of yoga and the one generally taught
in classes. 'Hatha' means force or will, and this branch
of yoga is therefore known as the yoga of will. The
student of hatha yoga gains mastery over their body
through practising the postures (*asanas*) and through
breath control (*pranayama*). Once the body is under
control, the student can turn their attention to gaining
control over the mind by meditation. When this has
been achieved, they are ready to proceed along the
eightfold path and join the path of Raja yoga (*see p.
184*). But most of us are content to stay with the postures and breathing to gain a better sense of wellbeing.

WHAT'S THE DIFFERENCE BETWEEN YOGA AND PHYSICAL EXERCISE?

Physical exercise aims primarily to tone the body, building strength, stamina and flexibility through exercise; the mind does not have to be engaged. Purely physical exercises can be done almost without thinking, even while listening to music or watching TV. And there is not always a sense of balance: for instance, a backbend might not be counterbalanced by a forward bend, resulting in a potential distortion in the body. Muscle bulk is built up without taking flexibility into consideration. And often physical exercises target one specific area without being applied to the body as a whole.

Yoga encompasses both body and mind. Although the *asanas* are physical postures, they must be approached with concentration and awareness. They are not just a means to physical fitness: they also lead to a well-balanced, flexible body and a clear mind. Breath control is also important. In all, harnessing of the body leads to harnessing of the mind, letting the student go on to pursue the spiritual side of yoga if they choose.

THE POSTURES

Each posture should be approached as though you are doing it for the first time – it is not like doing 100 press-ups. Both mind and body are involved. There should be no anticipation, otherwise it becomes purely automatic and you lose awareness of what your body is doing. You should take stock of how you feel, how your breath comes and goes; nothing should be rushed. Nor should you look around in class to see how anyone else is doing. Yoga is not competitive, it is about discovering your own body and yourself. You should concentrate on doing just as much of the posture as you are able, without forcing.

YOGA IS IDEAL FOR ALL AGES AND STAGES

- **Children**: Although youngsters are naturally supple, postures can help them build concentration
- **Stress sufferers**: Breathing and relaxation techniques are beneficial in coping with stress
- **Pregnant women**: Yoga can help prepare for birth – postures are adaptable for most stages and breathing techniques can help in labour
- **Disabled**: Many postures can be adapted to suit special needs without losing any of the benefits
- **Overweight**: Regular, gentle practise increases your feeling of wellbeing and enourages a more balanced approach to life and food. Many of the postures work on regulating the thyroid gland which dictates how your body uses up food.
- **Seniors**: The gentle approach to the postures lends itself to those of more advanced years and regular practice improves all-over flexibility.

DO YOU NEED TO BE YOUNG, THIN OR FIT TO START YOGA?

One of the great things about yoga is that anyone can take it up and benefit from it. You might be very stiff and wonder how you will ever manage a seated forward bend. The answer is you must only do as much as your body allows. In quite a short time and with regular practice you will find yourself becoming more supple and things you found impossible in your first class come more and more within your grasp. Yoga is not about comparing yourself to others in the class – even if they look as though they can bend in two!

WHAT BENEFITS ARE THERE?

The benefits of hatha yoga, working on both body and mind, cannot be underestimated. Compare a depressed person, often weighed down by worry, with shoulders and neck tensed and hunched. They may find it difficult to concentrate or make decisions. They have no energy and tend to neglect their bodies. On the other hand, a happy person walks with bright eyes, a spring in their step, their shoulders relaxed and wide, their spine straight. Their minds are focused on what they are doing and they have no problems making decisions. Yoga promotes this feeling of wellbeing by toning both the body and the mind.

The postures do not just work to tone and reshape the outside of the body, they also stimulate the internal organs and revitalise the nervous system.

THE PHYSICAL BENEFITS OF YOGA

- Creates energy and improves stamina, fitness and concentration
- Increases awareness of your body
- Keeps the body flexible so energy flows freely
- Works on internal organs and the endocrine system, and regulates metabolism
- Improves digestive and elimination processes
- Rejuvenates, decreases tension and teaches relaxation
- Improves posture and delays the ageing process
- Helps reduce excess fat
- Improves circulation and skin tone
- Can be done by all: young, old, male and female
- Needs no expensive equipment to practise
- Postures provide a full, balanced range of motion

THE MENTAL BENEFITS OF YOGA

- Calms and disciplines the mind
- Improves concentration and counteracts stress
- Gives control over emotions, particularly anger
- Creates a flexible mind where energy flows freely
- Promotes a positive, happy attitude

THE SPINE

You are as old as your spine is flexible, and in yoga particular attention is paid to the spine. The spine houses the spinal cord which carries instructions from the brain to the rest of the body and it is important to keep it in good working order. The normal adult spine has four gentle curves which protect the spine from any jarring. Many *asanas* work on the spine by bending it forward, backward and through twisting movements. The spinal-flexing exercises ensure the nerves get a good blood supply and there is none of the tension which often leads to back problems. Any vertebral irregularity is realigned by the twisting postures.

THE ENDOCRINE SYSTEM

This system controls the glands and hormones in the body. A healthy endocrine system is vital as it can affect our appearance, disposition and behaviour. Growth, body shape and the way in which the body uses food are also influenced by the endocrine system.

A person with a healthy endocrine system is usually strong, energetic, mentally alert and generally happy. A person whose endocrine system is not working properly may suffer from depression, obesity, sluggishness and fear. Women are often prone to ovarian problems while men may suffer from a lack of virility.

Specific postures work on different glands, mainly by increasing the blood supply to them. This increased blood supply brings with it oxygen and nutrients vital

for ensuring the glands' healthy working. To understand the benefits yoga postures bring, it helps to be
aware of the main glands in our body – where they
and what they do. A well-balanced yoga routine
should ensure the smooth running of all these gland

Pituitary gland At the base of the brain, it is known
the master gland. It regulates the growth of the enti
body and the development and functioning of the s
glands. The inverted (upside down) poses bring blo
to the brain and stimulate the pituitary gland.

Thyroid gland At the base of the neck, it controls
body growth and metabolism – the rate at which the

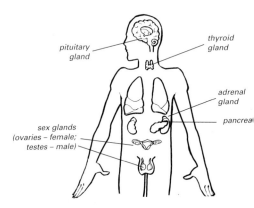

pituitary gland

thyroid gland

adrenal gland

pancrea

sex glands
(ovaries – female;
testes – male)

body uses food and oxygen. A sluggish thyroid gland slows a person down physically and mentally so they become lethargic and tend to gain weight easily. The inverted postures where the chin presses into the neck, stimulate and regulate this gland most effectively.

Pancreas Below the stomach, its function is to release substances which break down foodstuffs to aid digestion. It also regulates the level of sugar in the blood.

Adrenal glands Above the kidneys, these produce adrenalin. This hormone is released in conditions of stress and causes increased heartbeat, breathing, etc.

Sex glands Ovaries in women, testes in men. Their working is vital in developing gender characteristics.

WHY ARE THE POSTURES SO SPECIAL?

As already explained, the postures are known as *asanas* (pronounced _a_-sanas) in the Sanskrit. *Asana* means steady pose – once mastered, the postures are meant to be held steady for some time (although this is generally done by advanced students). When you practise yoga you will hear the postures' Sanskrit names used as well as their translations. It is useful to know both as many teachers, especially of the Iyengar method (see p. 20), use the Sanskrit, as do many yoga books. It may seem daunting at first but it won't take long to remember them. We have listed both English and Sanskrit names in a glossary at the back of the book (see p. 189).

It may be that some people are put off yoga because of

the Sanskrit names: the foreign language and strang
words can seem confusing. To ease yourself over an
difficulty, it is worth remembering that the names o
the postures usually refer to an animal (locust, cobr
cat) or a shape (triangle, bridge, half moon). Keep
meanings in mind when doing the posture so you h
an overall image of what the posture should look lik

The postures are not just a random series of movements: each has been carefully studied and develop
to help promote a healthy body and balanced mind
And balance is the key to yoga. Postures are done s
that they put the body through the whole range of
movements. In class a bend to the right will always
counterbalanced by a bend to the left; a backbend
be followed by a forward bend; and a twist to the le
will be followed by a twist to the right. A good teac
always presents a well-balanced class where the sele
tion of postures leaves you refreshed and revitalise
not exhausted and drained of energy. You should
always aim for this balance when practising at hom
Chapter 3 deals with the postures in more detail.

WHY IS BREATHING IMPORTANT?

Breathing is vital in yoga. Control of the breath lea
to control of the mind and it is this which distingu
es yoga from purely physical exercise. It is so important that a yogin – a master of yoga – measures
life not in years but in the number of breaths allott
for his lifetime. If he breathes hurriedly he squand
his time on earth.

Most of us are guilty of hardly breathing at all, tending to use perhaps a third of our lung capacity, at the top of the lungs. The ribcage scarcely moves and breathing tends to be quite fast and shallow, so we take in very little air which is so essential to the health of the body and internal organs. Breathing should involve the upper lungs (beneath the collarbones), the middle part where the ribcage expands, and the bottom section. Breathing into this bottom section is known as abdominal breathing, and brings the maximum amount of air to the largest area of the lungs. This breathing is slow and deep. Breathing should be done through the nose. Nostril hairs filter dust particles and the mucous lining helps kill germs. As air travels up the nasal passages it is warmed, ready to be taken into the lungs. If you breathe through your mouth all these benefits are lost.

BREATHING AND THE POSTURES

Awareness of breathing is important while undertaking the postures. Both the inhalation (breathing in) and exhalation (breathing out) are used to help the body into the pose. By paying special attention to the breath you can feel how it helps.

- **Inhalation** expands, lengthens and helps upward movements. It is used to lift out of the posture.
- **Exhalation** releases tension and helps downward movement. It is used to relax into a posture.

YOGA FOR YOU

WHY TAKE UP YOGA?

- To get fit
- To regulate weight
- To become more supple
- To help with back problems
- To learn how to relax
- To relieve stress
- To join an exercise class that is gentle
- To try something different

How to Learn: In Class or Self-Taught?

You may decide to learn yoga by yourself, perhaps from a book or a video. This is a good way to find out about yoga, but you should not underestimate the benefits of attending a class. The teacher is there to teach you the postures, and then make sure that you perform them correctly. A good teacher can spot imbalances – you might have your feet too close together or too far apart, or your bottom might be sticking out and throwing

out the whole balance and benefit of the posture. A
teacher talking you through a posture will bring out
its subtle aspects and make you aware of which parts
of your body are being stretched and which should be
relaxed. They will also talk you through the breathing.
It is difficult to be aware of all this practising on your
own. And the benefits of encouragement in a class are
very real. But it is important to find a style and a class
that suits you. It may take some time, but it is worth
looking around to see what is available in your area.

FINDING A CLASS

You can find out about yoga classes from a number of
sources. See **Useful Addresses** (*p. 188*) for associa-
tions listed here.

- The British Wheel of Yoga gives lists of local classes.

- In Scotland, the Scottish Yoga Teachers' Association
  publishes a list of hatha yoga classes.

- *Yoga & Health* magazine, published monthly in the
  UK, lists classes. Its classified ads also feature classes
  and courses in the UK, and yoga holidays abroad.

- On the Internet you can find out more about different schools of yoga and the teaching they offer.
  Many yoga sites also provide information on all the
  different aspects, with illustrated examples of the
  postures and step-by-step instructions.

- Many local authorities and leisure centres offer
  classes. Leisure centres often have mats so you

don't have to take one. In some private classes you
pay for a session which can last four or six weeks.

- Health-food shops, alternative bookshops and local
  shops may have notice boards with details of classes.
- Local libraries carry local-class information.

PRACTICAL CONSIDERATIONS

Should I consult a doctor first? You may have a medical condition which you need to take advice on
before joining a class.

Is there a class near you? Is it easy to get to, or
would you have to depend on public transport? Going
out on a cold winter's night can be very unappealing!

Is the class at a convenient time? Lunchtime classes
sound convenient but will you have to rush from work,
get changed then rush back? You could end up feeling
more stressed than relaxed. An evening class may start
too early to let you get home, eat and go out again. You
should always leave at least an hour and a half after
eating a light meal. And would an evening class finish
so late that you would almost be asleep by the end?

How long is the class? Ideally a class should be about
an hour and a half. One hour is quite short and there
may not be enough time for you to relax at the end.

Is it being held somewhere you feel comfortable?
Check the venue. It might be held in a cold, draughty
church hall. On the other hand, a leisure centre might
be quite noisy with other classes going on around you.

Is the yoga being taught the right approach for you?
The style often depends on the teacher. Yoga is physical, mental and spiritual. Many teachers develop a particular slant, emphasising one aspect over another. Ideally you will find a teacher who offers a balanced class that you feel comfortable in.

DIFFERENT TYPES OF YOGA TEACHING

Hatha yoga has developed, particularly as it has been introduced to the West. Teachers have brought their personal styles and attracted their own followings. Although all work with the same basic postures, they have adapted them to suit their individual approaches. There are five other styles you may come across.

Iyengar Yoga Based on the teachings of B K S Iyengar, this style of yoga is vigorous and includes the use of a variety of props – blocks (both foam and wooden), chairs and belts. A great deal of attention is paid to the details of the postures and students

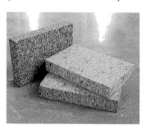

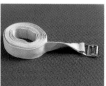

Typical props of Iyengar yoga: blocks and belt

progress from beginners to advanced. Students are taught to jump into the standing poses. Iyengar teachers undergo an Iyengar teacher-training course to qualify. You should be able to obtain a list of teachers in your area (*see* **Useful Addresses** *p. 188*).

Kundalini Yoga This aims to bring forth the energy, *kundalini*, stored at the base of the spine. It travels up the spine to the crown of the head. The postures and breathing techniques clear the way for this energy to travel. Chanting and meditation also play a part in arousing the energy. (*See* **Useful Addresses** *p. 188*.)

Astanga Yoga or Power Yoga This has become increasingly popular. It calls for strength, flexibility and stamina. Postures are done in a series linked by the breath. This type of yoga aims to strengthen and purify the nervous system, allowing energy, *prana*, to flow up through the spine. (*See* **Useful Addresses** *p. 188*.)

Viniyoga Developed by T K V Desikachar, this style works with breath, movement, sound, ritual and meditation. Attention is focused on the spine and postures are tailored to suit the needs of the individual student. Each person has their own physical, emotional and mental make-up so teaching is person-centred and taught one-to-one. (*See* **Useful Addresses** *p. 188*.)

Sivananda Yoga This style, founded by Swami Vishnu-Devananda, combines all the paths of yoga – *asana*, *pranayama*, selfless service, prayer, chanting, meditation and self-study. (*See* **Useful Addresses** *p. 188*.)

The Importance of a Good Teacher

It is important to find a good qualified teacher for you
to appreciate the benefits of yoga and to keep you
interested and motivated. A good teacher will also
make sure that you are doing the postures correctly –
something you cannot learn from a book or video.

A GOOD TEACHER ...

- gives a varied and balanced class
- judges the mood of the class and adjusts the class plan to suit it
- develops the postures over a number of weeks
- keeps the students motivated
- can explain the postures and make you aware of what you should feel when you do each one
- can explain clearly how the posture works on the body and describe the benefits
- observes students and rectifies faults in a positive, non-critical way. If they need to touch the student, this is done very gently with very little actual pressure
- warns who ought not to try a posture, e.g. high blood pressure sufferers, those menstruating
- can modify postures for students with specific problems or conditions, e.g. neck, back, physical disability, arthritis or pregnancy

What to Wear and Equipment to Take

The good thing about yoga is that you need practically no equipment. You should wear comfortable clothing – leggings and a tee-shirt or leotard and footless tights. But don't wear anything too baggy – the teacher needs to be able to see what your arms and legs are doing to check that you are performing the posture correctly. Don't wear socks: your bare feet will give a good grip on the floor and maximum awareness coming through the soles of your feet. And don't wear your watch as it can be distracting. Take a jumper or fleece and a pair of socks to wear during the relaxation session when your body cools down very quickly.

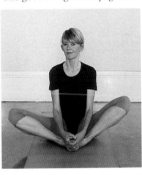

Ideal comfortable yoga wear

A non-slip mat is also very useful, letting you do the standing postures without slipping, and providing a firm base for the standing and balance postures. The teacher will be able to tell you where you can buy one and may be able to order it for you. They are also sold through classified ads of the monthly *Yoga & Health*.

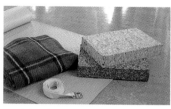

Mat, belt, blanket and blocks

You should also take a blanket (a plaid is ideal). It can be used for the seated and lying-down postures. You can also fold it up and use it for seated postures where you need to prop your hip up on one side. It also keeps you warm during the relaxation period at the end of the class. Try to keep the blanket solely for yoga practice.

Some teachers use foam blocks. They are useful to put under your buttocks when you are sitting with crossed legs and your knees should ideally be touching the ground. Blocks can also be used for support if you need to put your hand on the ground but cannot quite reach.

WHAT TO EXPECT IN CLASS

Classes tend to be predominantly female for hatha yoga, with more men attending Iyengar and Astanga (Power) yoga classes. However, this should not put anyone off from attending the type of class they pre-fer. For example, hatha yoga may look a very slow activity but the postures require strength and it can benefit men, who are often strong but lack suppleness.

The size of a class can vary from five to 30 people. There must be enough room for people to lie down and be able to stretch their arms out to the side. The teacher explains each posture and demonstrates it before the class attempts it. The teacher then talks th class through, observing each of the students to mak sure they are doing the posture correctly.

A well-structured class generally consists of:

- A warming-up session: perhaps including the cleansing and complete breaths
- A series of balanced postures: promoting stamina, strength, balance, suppleness, and a quiet mind
- A mix of postures: standing, seated, balancing, backbends, twists, inverted postures
- Relaxation

Attending a yoga class should leave you feeling balanced and better physically, mentally and emotionall

HOW TO BE A GOOD STUDENT

Yoga offers so much that it is worth putting in as mu effort as possible. See over for pointers to success.

Success depends on a cheerful disposition, persever-ance, courage, self-knowledge, unshakable faith in the word of the guru (teacher) and the avoidance of all superfluous company
Hatha Yoga Pradipika

SUCCESS IN YOGA

- Try to attend classes regularly
- Listen to the teacher; chatting is very distracting
- Don't anticipate the instructions. Come to each posture as though for the first time and be aware of how each part of your body is reacting
- Don't force it – only go as far as your body allows. Pain is the body's way of telling you this
- Pay attention to your breath. Use it to surrender into the pose. Inhaling is for energy, exhaling is for relaxing
- Concentrate fully on doing the postures, putting aside any worries and problems. You want your mind and emotions under control
- Practise the postures at home
- Be open to new ideas that the teacher offers

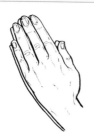

*Namasti –
the traditional form of
greeting in India and
used in yoga classes*

*'Om shanti, shanti,
shanti'*

*(Om = universal truth
Shanti = peace)*

THE POSTURES

Although there are reputed to be over 840,000 postures (believed to represent the total number of species of living beings), modern hatha yoga teaching puts the figure at around 200. But one 17th-century manual on the subject says there are 32 postures that are useful to human beings – a much more manageable number for the average yoga student! They have been carefully evolved through centuries to give a complete workout to the entire body, externally and internally, exercising every muscle, joint, nerve and gland. Practising them should secure a strong, flexible, healthy body. The yoga student can banish fatigue and should not be troubled by nervous disorders.

Many postures are named after natural beings: birds (crane, eagle), insects (locust, scorpion), animals (dog, cobra), fish and plants (lotus, tree). The actual shape of the posture resembles its namesake. When you practise, try to keep in your mind's eye the form you are assuming.

Cobra pose

Countering the Effects of Modern Life

Although yoga is ancient, it offers lessons on how to cope with life in a fast age when we seem to be losing touch with our bodies. Nowadays both children and adults spend hours sitting at desks, often in front of computer screens. The longer we do this, the more we slouch, neck forward, shoulders rounded, letting the muscles of the spine slacken. Tension builds up in all these areas.

If you watch a six-month-old baby learning to sit, you can see how easily and naturally it sits up with a beautifully straight spine. But if you try to imitate this by

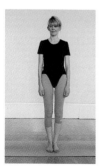

sitting on the floor, do you find your back becoming tired? You might feel some muscular discomfort and just long to let your spine collapse into its usual slump. The same may be true of how you stand. Good posture is something we lose over the years as age, gravity and habit take a hold. The basic standing posture, Mountain (*Tadasana*), teaches you how to stand correctly (*see left*).

Yoga postures go back to these very basic aspects and re-educate the body, making it aware of how it should really be feeling. Once you have learnt these basics, you will find it hard to ignore bad habits in the future. Even if you do give in to them, you will still be aware of them!

How Postures Balance & Complement Each Other

As has been mentioned before, yoga postures are not done individually. A balanced session should include a mixture of standing, lying, inverted, backbends, seated and balancing postures, and bear in mind some basic guidelines:

1 Always begin with a warming-up session to limber up and loosen the spine and joints.

2 Hold each posture for a few seconds. Rest for a moment or two between postures and move slowly and gracefully.

3 Don't include too many standing postures in a session. They promote strength and may enourage aggression. You should never push yourself too far, even trying to compete with what you have achieved before.

4 Balance forward bends with backward bends.

5 If you compress one part of the body in a posture, e.g. the front of the neck in Plough (*Halasana*), then you must extend it in a counterpose; e.g. in Fish (*Matsyasana*).

6 Always practise to each side in postures such as Triangle (*Trikonasana*) or the twists.

7 Leave stong backbends such as Cobra (*Bhujangasana*) or Locust (*Salabhasana*) until quite well into the session. Your spine and hips need time to loosen and limber up before tackling these.

8 End a session with a quietening, closing down pose such as Seated Forward Bend (*Paschimottanasana*).

9 Allow a few minutes' relaxation at the end of the session.

The Importance of Right Breathing

Please note that when we talk of breathing here we are not referring to *pranayama* or other yogic breathing techniques; these are discussed separately on page 164 in the chapter Yogic Breathing. Breathing in the context of *asana* is to raise energy and relax into the posture.

What makes yoga unique as an exercise system is that the breath plays a major part in how each posture is approached. The breath is used to explore and develop the postures. Breathing consists of the in-breath (inhalation) and the out-breath (exhalation). While performing the postures breathing should be done through the nose, unless otherwise advised.

Inhalation, which brings vital oxygen into the body, is energising. Generally, the in-breath is used to move the body into the posture; while exhalation, which removes impurities from the body, is used to relax into the posture.

Because breathing plays such an important part in yoga, it is important not to neglect it. This is especially

BREATHING

In-breath expands, lengthens and helps upward movement. For example, you would raise arms on an in-breath but lower them on an out-breath. You would use the in-breath to lift out of a seated forward bend.

Out-breath releases tension, and helps downward movement. For example, you would breathe out going into a seated forward bend. Once you were in the pose you would use another out-breath to relax further into the forward bend.

important when learning at home from a book or video. Pay attention to the breathing instructions for each posture – you will find that they help.

The importance of breathing correctly is another reason why it is advisable to try to attend a class.

Eye Exercises

> **CAUTION**
>
> The eye exercises should not be done while wearing contact lenses

1 Sit in a comfortable pose with your spine straight, shoulders relaxed and back, chin parallel to the floor and eyes looking straight ahead. Without moving the head, look diagonally up to the right as far as you can. Then look diagonally down to the left as far as you can. Repeat three times.
   Then do it in the opposite direction, looking diagonally up to the left and then diagonally down to the right. Repeat three times.

2 Without moving the head, look straight up towards the ceiling and then down to the floor. Repeat three times.

3 Without moving the head, look as far to the right as you can, then look as far to the left as you can. Repeat three times.

4 Move the eyes in a circular motion moving to the right (clockwise). You want to make the biggest circle as possible with your eyes. Repeat three times. Then do the same but circle to the left (anti-clockwise). Repeat three times.

5 Stretch your left arm out in front of you with the index finger pointing up. It should be at eye level. Take your right index finger and place it half way between the left finger and your eyes. Focus both eyes first of the farther left index finger, then focus both eyes on the closer right index finger. Repeat three times.

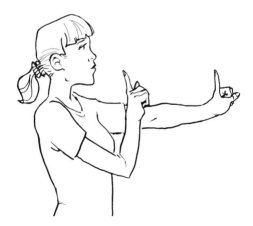

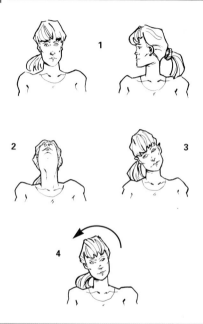

CAUTION

Take great care if you have any of these conditions:
osteoporosis, osteoarthrosis, arthritis, ear problems

Neck Exercises

1 Sit in a comfortable pose with your spine straight, shoulders relaxed and back, chin parallel to the floor, eyes looking straight ahead. Without moving your shoulders, turn your head as far as you can to the right, trying to look at the wall behind you. Then turn your head as far as you can to the left, making sure that the shoulders do not move. Repeat four times in each direction.

2 Keeping your shoulders still, drop your head forward to your chest, then take it up and back so that you are looking at the ceiling. Try not to scrunch the back of the neck, imagine you have a rolled-up towel wedged there. Repeat both movements four times.

3 With eyes looking straight ahead, drop your head sideways as though your right ear is trying to touch your right shoulder. Don't be tempted to lift the shoulder to meet the ear! Then repeat on the left side. Repeat four times on each side.

4 Let your head drop forward to your chest. Then roll head round to the right in a wide circular movement. Perform four entire circles to the right then repeat the same circular movement to the left. Take care not to move the shoulders during this exercise.

Butterfly

numbers correspond to instructions on p. 37

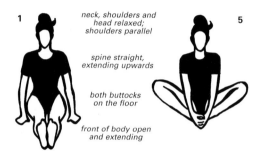

1

neck, shoulders and
head relaxed;
shoulders parallel

spine straight,
extending upwards

both buttocks
on the floor

front of body open
and extending

5

CAUTIONS

- Take care if you have knee or hip problems
- Do not push the knees down onto the floor with the hands

NOTE

Movement should flow; the legs represent the wings of a butterfly, fluttering up and down

BENEFITS

- Strengthens and stimulates leg muscles
- Tones thigh muscles
- Helpful for sciatic pain/lower-back pain
- Stimulates abdominal organs

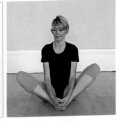

1 Sit in Rod or Staff (*p. 82*), basis of the sitting poses.

2 Bend knees out to sides, bringing soles of feet together in front of the body.

3 Clasp hands, interlinking fingers around toes of both feet, and draw heels close in towards crotch (keep outside edges of feet and little toes on floor).

4 Breathe in; stretch spine upwards from tailbone to top of head; open and expand the body.

5 Breathe out; push knees out and down, opening and stretching inner muscles of legs. Aim to bring outside of legs and knees onto floor.

6 Repeat a few times, using the breath. Breathe out; extend and stretch knees out to sides and down. Breathe in; relax knees and leg muscles.

Cat

numbers correspond to instructions on p. 39

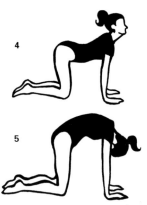

4

ensure arms are
straight

keep shoulders
relaxed and low

5

hips and shoulders
are parallel

CAUTIONS

- Approach with care if you have back problems
- Take care if you have knee or wrist problems

NOTE

Hands, knees and feet do not move in this posture;
only the spine and back move, flexing up and down

BENEFITS

- Brings flexibility to spine
- Strengthens back, arms
- Tones and firms buttock, hamstring muscles
- Stimulates nervous system
- Improves circulation, digestion

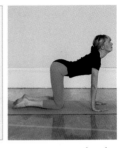

1 From a kneeling position, come up onto your hands and knees.

2 Place hands, palms down, directly below your shoulders, shoulder-width apart, arms straight and fingers pointing forward.

3 Place knees directly below hips, hip-width apart, with tops of feet rest on floor.

4 Breathe out; arch the back like an angry cat, pull abdominal muscles inward and upward, and tuck chin in towards chest.

5 Breathe in; drop tummy and abdominal muscles, concaving your lower back, raise head and look up (keep arms straight and shoulders low). Feel your buttocks spreading.

6 Repeat a few times in a flowing movement, using the breath.

Pelvic Lift

numbers correspond to instructions on p. 41

3

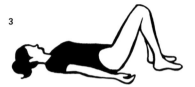

shoulders and feet parallel
pelvis and front of body push upwards
feet and legs hip-width apart
toes point directly forward
soles of the feet push down into the floor

5

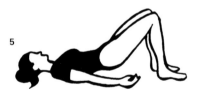

CAUTIONS

- Take care if you have abdominal problems
- Approach with care if you have back or knee problems

BENEFITS

- Tones thighs, hips, buttocks
- Strengthens legs, lower back
- Stimulates abdominal organs
- Opens front of body

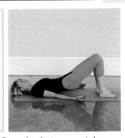

1 Lie with back flat on the floor, body in a straight line. Relax arms by sides.

2 Bend knees and put soles of feet flat on floor. Bring heels close in towards buttocks, feet hip-width apart; toes point forward and knees point up to ceiling.

3 Relax arms by sides, in line with shoulders; turn palms to face the ceiling.

4 Breathe in; raise buttocks 4 to 6 in off the floor, tighten thigh and buttock muscles and push pelvis up towards the ceiling, knees pointing upwards (feel lower back raise up off the floor). Chin is tucked in.

5 Breathe out; push hands into floor and, with back of head on floor, slowly uncurl spine (top to bottom) onto floor.

6 Repeat several times, raising up on the in-breath and lowering on the out-breath.

Salute to the Sun
(*Surya Namaskar*)

A series of 12 postures practised in a flowing sequence combining the use of the breath.

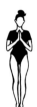

1
body straight;
weight even
on both feet;
head, neck,
shoulders
relaxed;
elbows close
in by body

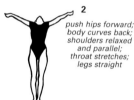

2
push hips forward;
body curves back;
shoulders relaxed
and parallel;
throat stretches;
legs straight

3
legs straight,
knees back;
shoulders
relaxed, parallel;
top of head
faces floor;
push tailbone up

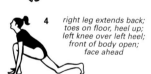

4
right leg extends back;
toes on floor, heel up;
left knee over left heel;
front of body open;
face ahead

CAUTIONS

- Do not practise if you have severe arthritis
- Be careful if you have stiff joints or back problems
- Approach with caution if you have high or low blood pressure

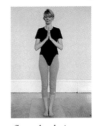

BENEFITS

- Stimulates and ener-
  gises the whole body
- Improves circulation
- Strengthens arms, legs
- Increases spine flexi-
  bility and suppleness

1 Stand, feet together and flat on floor, body in a
   straight line facing forward (Mountain; see p. 48).
   Bring the hands into Namasti (prayer position; see
   p. 26) at mid-chest; fingers point to ceiling.

2 Breathe in; stretch arms up and arch the body back
   from hips; keep arms shoulder-width apart, palms
   forward. Drop head back and look at the ceiling.

3 Breathe out; extend the body and arms forward,
   hingeing at hips, and bring palms down onto floor
   at outside of feet; fingers point forward. Bring
   abdomen and chest in towards thighs, forehead to
   shins. Tuck chin in towards chest; top of the head
   faces the floor. (Standing Forward Bend; see p. 70.)

4 Breathe in; raise head and chest and look forward.
   Stretch right leg back as far as possible, bend right
   knee and place it on the floor. Tuck right toes
   under, heel points to the ceiling. Simultaneously
   bend the left knee, place it directly above left heel.
   Left thigh is parallel to floor, sole of left foot is flat
   on the floor.

Salute to the Sun
(continued)

5 *legs straight; arms straight; hips and shoulders parallel; head and neck relaxed; top of head pushing to floor; tailbone pushing to ceiling; buttocks wide*

6 *toes, knees, chest and chin on floor; stomach off the floor; hips and shoulders parallel; arms and elbows close in beside body*

7 *front of body open, expanding; weight on hands and toes; shoulders and hips parallel; neck and head relaxed; face looks upwards*

8
instructions are as for 5

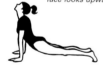

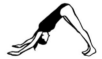

CAUTIONS

- Do not practise if you have severe arthritis
- Be careful if you have stiff joints or back problems
- Approach with caution if you have high or low blood pressure

BENEFITS

- Increases joint movement and flexibility: ankles, knees, hips, wrists, elbows, shoulders
- Opens and expands the chest

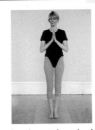

5 Breathe out; stretch left leg back, place it beside the right. Push heels down to floor, pull kneecaps up. Push backs of legs up to ceiling, stretching them fully. Simultaneously stretch arms out fully in front of body. Push palms and heels down to floor, extend tailbone up to the ceiling and spread buttocks wide. (Downward-Facing Dog; see p. 144.)

6 Push weight onto palms and toes, lower the body; bring knees, chest and chin onto floor; face forward.

7 Breathe in; straighten arms and pull the body and legs forward, bringing chest through in front of arms. Drop head back and look up to the ceiling. (Upward-Facing Dog; see p. 124.)

8 Breathe out; push hips and tailbone up to the ceiling. Push thighs back, out of the hips, pull up kneecaps, push heels down to the floor. Feel legs straighten and stretch. Extend the body from the hips down towards the floor; top of head faces the floor. Push tailbone up towards the ceiling, spread buttocks wide. (Downward-Facing Dog; see p. 144.)

Salute to the Sun
(*continued*)

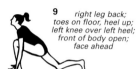

9 right leg back;
toes on floor, heel up;
left knee over left heel;
front of body open;
face ahead

10 legs straight,
knees back;
shoulders
relaxed, parallel;
top of head
faces floor;
tailbone up

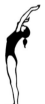

11
push hips forward;
body curves back;
shoulders relaxed
and parallel;
throat stretches;
legs straight

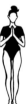

12
body straight;
weight even on
both feet;
head, neck and
shoulders
relaxed;
elbows close in
by body

CAUTIONS

- Do not practise if you have severe arthritis
- Be careful if you have stiff joints or back problems
- Approach with caution if you have high or low blood pressure

BENEFITS

- Relieves and releases upper-body congestion
- Tones and stimulates the internal organs
- Helpful for back pain

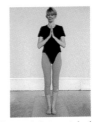

9 Breathe in; raise head, look forward, bring right leg forward and place sole of foot on floor, between palms, toes pointing forward. (Right knee is above right heel, right thigh parallel to the floor. Left leg is stretched out behind, knees and toes on floor.)

10 Breathe out; bring left leg forward to place left foot flat beside right foot, toes forward. Straighten legs, pull up kneecaps and bring front of body in close to legs. Place palms down on floor beside feet, fingers forward. (Standing Forward Bend; see p. 70.)

11 Breathe in; raise body and arms to vertical, bring arms over head, shoulder-width apart, palms forward. Arch body back at hips, drop head back and look up to ceiling.

12 Breathe out; bring body and arms to vertical, lower arms and bring hands into Namasti at mid-chest, fingers pointing to ceiling. Body is in start position.

13 Repeat the sequence to other side; left leg back first. Then repeat the sequence a few times, to each side.

Mountain
(*Tadasana*)

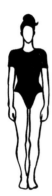

*chin points down
towards the floor*

back of neck is long

*relaxed shoulders
and arms*

*hips and shoulders
face forward*

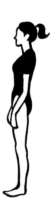

NOTES

Ensure the body weight is evenly distributed
across the soles of both feet. This posture should
be practised before and after all standing postures.
In Tadasana the body is rooted to the ground and
is steady like a mountain.

BENEFITS

- Encourages good posture
- Helps realign and balance the body
- Allows body to become calm

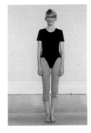

1 Stand with feet together flat on the floor, big toe joints and inner ankle bones slightly touching, toes pointing forward.
2 Hold body in a straight line, facing forward. Relax arms down by sides, palms facing in towards body with fingers gently curled; thumbnails face forward.
3 Pull kneecaps up and lift up leg muscles and bones.
4 Tuck tailbone under.
5 Lift up and open front of body.
6 Relax shoulders down and lengthen back of neck by lowering chin slightly. Rest head evenly at top of spine. Maintain a straight upright posture, hold and breathe normally.

Tree
(*Vrksasana*)
numbers correspond to instructions on p. 51

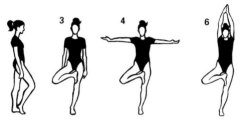

hips and shoulders are parallel
extended knee stretches out to the side, not forward
arms are straight and upper arms hug ears

CAUTIONS

- Do not come out of the posture quickly
- Take care if you have ankle or knee problems
- Approach with care if you suffer from vertigo
  (use a wall as a support behind you)

NOTES

Concentrate on a fixed spot on the floor in front of
you to help you balance.

BENEFITS

- Promotes good posture
- Aids concentration
- Improves balance and co-ordination
- Strengthens leg muscles

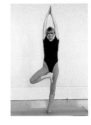

1 Stand in Mountain (*p. 48*), basis of the standing poses.

2 Bend right knee up to chest, take right foot and put sole high up against inner left thigh. Aim right heel for the crotch and push heel in towards left thigh, right toes pointing to floor. Right knee extends to side. (Feel stretch in right thigh; hips opening out.)

3 Keep left leg straight, pulling kneecap up (feel left leg strong).

4 Breathe in; raise arms out by sides to shoulder level, palms face up. Breathe out.

5 Breathe in; raise arms, straight, above head and bring palms together. Breathe out.

6 Stretch and extend body upwards from left foot to fingertips, lifting and opening out at front of body. Hold and breathe normally in the posture.

7 Lower arms down by sides, release right foot and replace it on the floor beside left foot.

8 Repeat the posture to the other side.

Triangle
(*Trikonasana*)
numbers correspond to instructions on p. 53

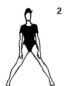
2

3

4

legs are straight
front and side of body
open out
shoulders relaxed
neck long
hips and shoulders
face forward

5

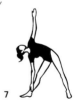
7

CAUTIONS

- Take care if you have knee problems
- Take care if you have arthritic hips

BENEFITS

- Tones leg, buttock muscles
- Encourages flexibility in hips
- Opens chest
- Helps digestive problems

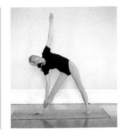

1 Stand in Mountain (*p. 48*), basis of the standing poses.

2 Take feet 3 to 3.5 ft apart.

3 Turn right foot out to a 90° angle and left foot in to 45° (right heel is in line with left instep).

4 Breathe in; stretch up spine and raise both arms to shoulder level (palms face down).

5 Breathe out; extend right arm out to side, bring right hand down right leg towards the floor, palm facing forward (feel the stretch along left side of body).

6 Breathe in; raise left arm up to vertical (palm forward). Feel chest open and expand.

7 Breathe out; turn head up towards left hand (aim to have a straight line from top hand to bottom hand).

8 Turn head to look forward, raise body up to vertical, arms outstretched at shoulder level. Breathe out; relax arms down by sides, feet face forward.

9 Repeat from step 3 to the other side.

Flank Stretch
(*Parsvakonasana*)
numbers correspond to instructions on p. 55 and 57

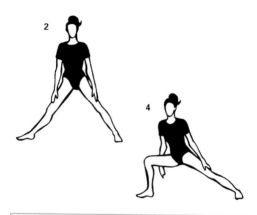

2

4

CAUTIONS

- Approach with care if you have hip or back problems
- If you have neck or shoulder problems, keep the top arm relaxed along the side of the body

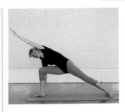

1 Stand in Mountain (*p. 48*), basis of the standing poses.

2 Take feet 4 to 4.5 ft apart. Turn right foot out to a 90° angle and left foot in to 45° (right heel is in line with left instep).

3 Breathe in; raise arms out to shoulder level, palms facing the floor.

4 Bend right knee and put it directly above right heel, thigh parallel with floor (aim to have a 90° angle at knee). Extend the body to the right and rest right forearm on top of right thigh; body and face forward.

5 Breathe in; raise left arm up to the vertical; reach for the ceiling and take it towards left ear. (Feel the stretch along left side, and right side come closer to right thigh.)

continued on p. 57

Flank Stretch
(*continued*)

6

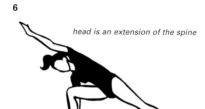

head is an extension of the spine

right angle at right knee joint
tailbone and right thigh push down to the floor

left arm straight
left leg straight
straight line along left side of the body

CAUTIONS

- Approach with care if you have hip or back problems

- If you have neck or shoulder problems, keep the top arm relaxed along the side of the body

BENEFITS

- Strengthens feet, legs
- Helps with hip and lower-back problems
- Stimulates digestion
- Helpful for respiratory problems

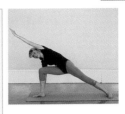

continued from p. 55

6 Breathe out; place palm of right hand onto floor at outside of right foot, fingers pointing in the same direction as right toes. Bring right side of body forward, roll left side back and up towards the ceiling. (Feel the diagonal stretch along the left side of body, from outer ankle to fingertips.) Hold the posture and breathe normally.

7 Breathe in; straighten right leg and raise body up to vertical. Extend arms out by sides at shoulder level. Breathe out; relax arms down by sides, turn toes to point forward.

8 Repeat the posture to the other side from step 2.

Warrior I
(*Virabhadrasana I*)
numbers correspond to instructions on pages 59 & 61

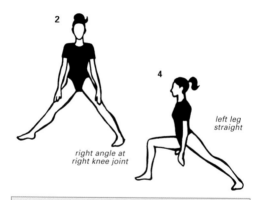

2

*right angle at
right knee joint*

4

*left leg
straight*

CAUTIONS

- Do not attempt if you have a slipped disc
- Do not take arms above head if you have high or low blood pressure (relax arms down by sides)
- Approach with care if you have back, hip or shoulder problems

BENEFITS

- Strengthens legs
- Strengthens ankle, knee joints
- Helps develop the chest
- Helpful for sciatica
- Stimulates 'inner' strength

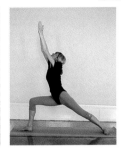

1 Stand in Mountain (*p. 48*), basis of the standing poses.

2 Take feet 4 to 4.5 ft apart. Turn right foot out to a 90° angle and left foot in to 45° (right heel is in line with left instep).

3 Breathe out; rotate hips and turn body around to the right (with front of body facing in the same direction as right toes).

4 Bend right knee and place it directly above right heel, with right thigh parallel to the floor and right knee pointing directly towards right toes (make a right angle at right-knee joint). Left leg is straight, push soles of both feet into the floor.

5 Breathe in; raise arms above head, keeping them straight and shoulder-width apart with palms facing. Stretch arms up, fingertips reaching for the ceiling.

continues on p. 61

Warrior I
(*continued*)

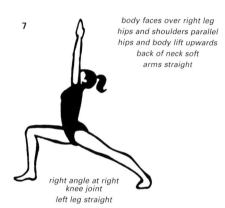

7

body faces over right leg
hips and shoulders parallel
hips and body lift upwards
back of neck soft
arms straight

right angle at right
knee joint
left leg straight

CAUTIONS

- Do not attempt if you have a slipped disc
- Do not take arms above head if you have high or low blood pressure (relax arms down by sides)
- Approach with care if you have back, hip or shoulder problems

BENEFITS

- Strengthens legs
- Strengthens ankle, knee joints
- Helps develop the chest
- Helpful for sciatica
- Stimulates 'inner' strength

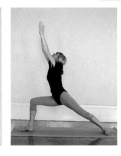

continues from p. 59

6 Breathe out; slowly drop head back and look up between palms to the ceiling. Hold the posture and breathe normally. The back of the neck should be soft.

7 Breathe in, raise head to vertical; breathe out, straighten right leg, turn body to the front, relax arms down by sides, turn toes to point forward.

8 Keeping feet wide, repeat to the other side from step 2.

Warrior II
(*Virabhadrasana II*)

numbers correspond to instructions on pages 63 & 65

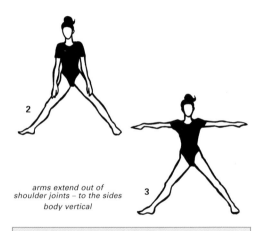

arms extend out of shoulder joints – to the sides
body vertical

CAUTIONS

- Take care if you have arthritic hips
- Approach with caution if you have ankle or knee problems

BENEFITS

- Opens and expands chest – encourages deep breathing
- Stimulates abdominal organs
- Stimulates 'inner' strength

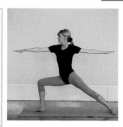

1 Stand in Mountain (*p. 48*), basis of the standing poses.

2 Take feet 4 to 4.5 ft apart. Turn right foot out to a 90° angle and left foot in to 45° (right heel is in line with left instep).

3 Breathe in; extend arms out to sides at shoulder level, palms facing floor and body facing forward.

4 Breathe out; bend right knee and place it directly above right heel, with right thigh parallel to the floor (make a right angle at the right knee joint). Left leg is straight; push soles of both feet into the floor.

5 Breathe in; extend and stretch body upwards from tailbone to top of head. Open and expand body – front chest and ribcage expand out to the sides. Keep hips and shoulders parallel.

continues on p. 65

Warrior II
(continued)

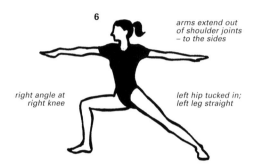

6

arms extend out
of shoulder joints
– to the sides

right angle at
right knee

left hip tucked in;
left leg straight

body vertical
soles of the feet pushing down into the floor

CAUTIONS

- Take care if you have arthritic hips
- Approach with caution if you have ankle or knee
  problems

BENEFITS

• Encourages greater-flexibility in hips and shoulders

• Helpful for upper-back and shoulder pain

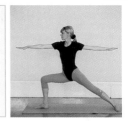

continued from p. 63

6 Breathe out; turn the head to the right and look towards fingertips of right hand. Keep shoulders low and relaxed, body facing forward. Hold the posture and breathe normally.

7 Breathe in; straighten right leg. Breathe out, turn head and toes to point forward; relax the arms down by sides.

8 Keeping feet wide, repeat to the other side from step 2.

Half Moon
(*Ardha Chandrasana*)

numbers correspond to instructions on pages 67 & 69

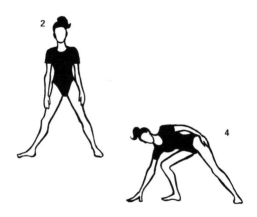

CAUTIONS

- Do not practise if you have arthritic hips
- If you feel unsteady in the posture, practise with your back against a wall

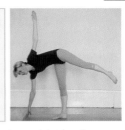

BENEFITS

- Encourages mobility in hips
- Opens and expands front of body
- Increases circulation to lower half of body

1 Stand in Mountain *(p. 48)*, basis of the standing poses.

2 Take feet 3 to 3.5 ft apart. Turn right foot out to a 90° angle and left foot in to 45° (right heel is in line with left instep).

3 Breathe in; raise arms out to shoulder level, palms facing floor. Bring right hand down towards right foot. Relax left arm and hand along left side; body faces forward.

4 Bend right knee and place right fingertips on floor, 12 in forward of right foot. Body faces forward, and face is looking straight ahead.

5 Breathe in; raise left leg straight up to horizontal in line with left hip; toes and knee face forward. Push left heel away from body, stretch left leg. Simultaneously straighten right leg.

continues on p. 69

Half Moon
(*continued*)

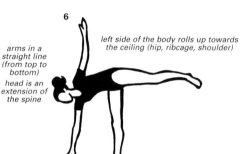

legs straight
arms straight
body faces forward

6

*left side of the body rolls up towards
the ceiling (hip, ribcage, shoulder)*

*arms in a
straight line
(from top to
bottom)*

*head is an
extension of
the spine*

CAUTIONS

- Do not practise if you have arthritic hips
- If you feel unsteady in the posture, practise with your back against a wall

BENEFITS

- Encourages mobility in hips
- Opens and expands front of body
- Increases circulation to lower half of body

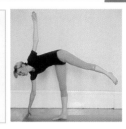

continues from p. 67

6 Breathe out; straighten right arm. The right hand does not bear weight – it is simply a support for balance. Raise left arm straight up to vertical, push fingertips up towards ceiling, palm faces forward (left arm in line with right arm). Bring the right side of the body forward, roll the left side of the body back and up towards the ceiling. Feel the front of the body open and expand. Hold the posture and breathe normally.

7 Bend right knee, stretch left leg back, put sole of left foot on floor. Straighten both legs. Breathe in; raise body to vertical, arms outstretched at shoulder level. Breathe out; relax arms down by sides, feet facing forward.

8 Repeat the posture to the other side from step 2.

Standing Forward Bend
(*Uttanasana*)
numbers correspond to instructions on pages 71 & 73

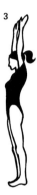

3

legs straight
relax back of neck and head
push shoulderblades down towards the waist
hips and shoulders parallel

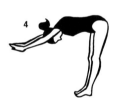

4

CAUTIONS

- Avoid forward bends if you have eye problems
- Do not attempt if you suffer from high or low blood pressure
- Approach with care if you have lower back pain or sciatica

BENEFITS

- Tones leg muscles
- Improves upper-body circulation
- Tones abdominal organs
- Calms yet energises the body

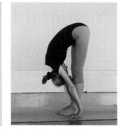

1 Stand in Mountain (*p. 48*), basis of the standing poses.

2 Take feet hip-width apart, feet parallel, toes pointing forward. Pull kneecaps up (feel legs strengthen and stretch).

3 Breathe in; stretch spine upwards from tailbone to top of head and raise arms straight above head, shoulder-width apart, palms facing.

4 Breathe out; extend body and arms forward, hingeing from hips. Lead with chest (to flatten the back) and bring chest and abdomen down onto front of thighs; place forehead onto shins.

5 Place palms of hands down on the floor beside feet, fingers pointing forward. Gently push palms into the floor and bring front of body close in to front of the legs, top of head facing floor.

continues on p. 73

Standing Forward Bend
(continued)

hips and shoulders parallel

6

*shoulderblades
push down
towards the
waist
back of neck and
head relaxed*

legs straight

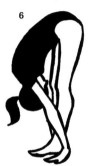

CAUTIONS

- Avoid forward bends if you have eye problems
- Do not attempt if you suffer from high or low blood pressure
- Approach with care if you have lower back pain or sciatica

BENEFITS

- Tones leg muscles
- Improves upper-body circulation
- Tones abdominal organs
- Calms yet energises the body

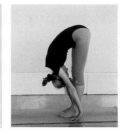

continues from p. 71

6 Hold the posture and breathe normally. (Feel the stretch up the legs, from heels to buttock bones, and feel spine extending downwards from tailbone to top of the head.)

7 To come out: bend knees, breathe in and raise body and arms to vertical. Breathe out, lower arms down by ankles and straighten legs.

NOTES

If your palms do not touch the floor, place them around the ankles or onto backs of legs, whichever is more comfortable. Keep legs straight and on each out-breath pull on the ankles or legs, extending the elbows out to sides; bring front of the body closer to the front of the legs.

Sideways Forward Bend

(*Parsvottanasana*)

numbers correspond to instructions on pages 75 & 77

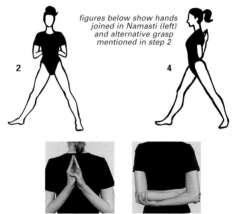

figures below show hands
joined in Namasti (left)
and alternative grasp
mentioned in step 2

2

4

CAUTIONS

- Do not do if you have high or low blood pressure
- Avoid forward bends if you have eye problems
- Take care if you have arthritic hips, shoulders or wrists

BENEFITS

- Relieves leg stiffness
- Brings flexibility to wrists, shoulders and hips
- Tones abdominal organs
- Helps correct 'rounded' shoulders

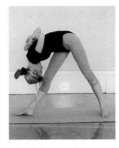

1 Stand in Mountain (*p. 48*), basis of the standing poses.

2 Bring palms of hands together into a prayer position (Namasti) behind back, hands in line with shoulder blades, outside edges of little fingers in contact with spine and fingers point to the ceiling. (If this is too difficult, bend your arms at the elbows behind your back and take hold of right elbow with left hand and left elbow with right.) See opposite page.

3 Take the feet 3 to 3.5 ft apart. Turn right foot out to a 90° angle and left foot in to 45° (right heel is in line with left instep).

4 Rotate body from hips round to the right, with front of the body facing forward in the same direction as right toes.

5 Breathe in; stretch spine up from tailbone to top of head. Open and expand the body.

continues on p. 77

Sideways Forward Bend
(*continued*)

elbows lift up towards the ceiling
hips and shoulders parallel
head relaxed

6

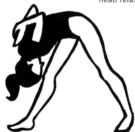

legs straight
weight pushed onto back foot
tailbone pushes up towards the ceiling

CAUTIONS

- Do not do if you have high or low blood pressure
- Avoid forward bends if you have eye problems
- Take care if you have arthritic hips, shoulders or wrists

BENEFITS

- Relieves leg stiffness
- Brings flexibility to wrists, shoulders and hips
- Tones abdominal organs
- Helps correct 'rounded' shoulders

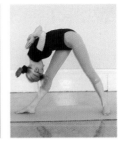

continues from p. 75

6 Breathe out; extend body forward from hips, lead with chin (to flatten the back) and stretch body down along right leg. Aim to place abdomen and chest on right thigh, and forehead on right shin. Lengthen spine and back of neck down towards the floor, with top of the head facing the floor; tuck chin in. Stretch elbows up towards the ceiling, keeping hands in Namasti. Hold the posture, breathing normally. On each out-breath, stretch and extend the body further down into the posture. Push tailbone up towards the ceiling, and widen buttocks.

7 Breathe in; raise head and body to the vertical; breathe out, turn body to the front, release hands and relax arms down by sides, turning the toes to point forward.

8 Repeat the posture to the other side from step 2.

Wide-Leg Forward Bend
(Prasarita Padottanasana)
numbers correspond to instructions on p. 79 and 81

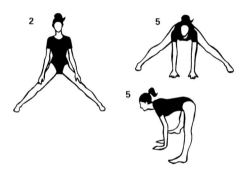

CAUTIONS

- Do not do if you have high or low blood pressure
- Avoid forward bends if you have eye problems
- Do not practice if you have a slipped disc
- Approach with care if you have head, ear or neck problems
- Go into the posture slowly, particularly if you have back problems

BENEFITS

- Opens and expands hips and chest
- Increases circulation in upper body
- Aids digestion
- Stretches leg and thigh muscles

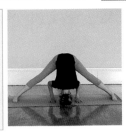

1 Stand in Mountain (*p. 48*), basis of the standing poses.

2 Take feet 4 to 4.5 ft apart, keeping them parallel with toes pointing forward. Pull kneecaps up, lift insteps (feel your legs strengthen).

3 Breathe in; extend spine upwards from tailbone to top of head. Lift and open front of body. Tuck tailbone under and forwards.

4 Breathe out; extend body forward, hingeing at hips. Lead with chest to flatten back, bring body to the horizontal (parallel with the floor). Place hands palms down onto the floor directly below shoulders with arms straight and fingers pointing forward.

5 Breathe in; raise head and look forward. Take hands back in line with feet, palms on floor, shoulder-width apart and fingers point forward.

continues on p. 81

Wide-Leg Forward Bend
(*continued*)

6

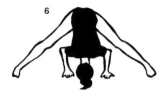

6

no weight on the head
arms at right angles below the body
back of body extending downwards
legs straight
soles of the feet flat on the floor
weight evenly distributed on hands
and feet

CAUTIONS

- Do not do if you have high or low blood pressure
- Avoid forward bends if you have eye problems
- Do not practise if you have a slipped disc
- Approach with care if you have head, ear or neck problems
- Go into the posture slowly, particularly if you have back problems

BENEFITS

- Opens and expands hips and chest
- Increases circulation in upper body
- Aids digestion
- Stretches leg and thigh muscles

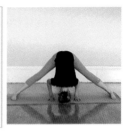

continues from p. 79

6 Breathe out; bend elbows back below body (making right angles with arms). Extend body and spine downwards and bring top of head down onto the floor, below body. Push palms into floor, keeping elbows bent, then lift shoulders and push tailbone up towards ceiling (feel your back extending). Breathe normally. On each out-breath stretch and extend the body further down into the posture.

7 Breathe in, raise head and body to the horizontal with arms straight and palms on floor below shoulders. Breathe out, move feet closer together by pointing in toes then heels until feet are together. Breathe in, raise body and head to vertical; breathe out, move toes and heels to bring feet together, relax arms down by sides.

Rod or Staff
(*Dandasana*)

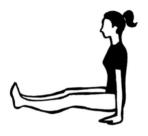

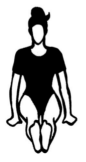

shoulders and hips parallel
shoulders relaxed
spine straight
legs straight
front of chest lifts and
opens
do not let the head tilt

BENEFITS

- Strengthens leg muscles
- Opens front chest
- Improves posture
- Brings about body awareness

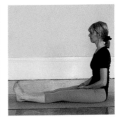

1 Sit tall on buttock bones, legs outstretched in front of the body, relaxing arms down by sides.

2 Bring legs together, inner ankle bones and inner knee joints touching. (If you find this difficult, have legs slightly apart.)

3 Push heels away from the body, toes point upwards.

4 Breathe in; straighten and stretch up through spine, from tailbone to top of head.

5 Breathe out; relax shoulders down, open and expand front of the body, keeping spine straight.

6 Relax arms by sides of the body, palms resting on the floor beside hips, fingers point forwards.

7 Lengthen back of the neck by lowering chin slightly; balance head evenly at top of spine, face looking forward. Maintain a straight upright posture, hold and breathe normally.

Hero
(*Virasana*)

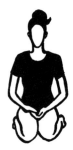

shoulders parallel
body stretches/extends upwards
buttocks flat on floor
toes point back

CAUTIONS

- Do not practise if you have knee or hip problems
- Do not practise if you have varicose veins

NOTES

- If the buttocks cannot come on to the floor between the feet, place a folded blanket/s below them, and rest the buttocks on the blanket/s

BENEFITS

- Stimulates leg muscles
- Opens chest, encourages deep breathing
- Helpful for respiratory problems
- Calms the whole body
- Beneficial for flat feet

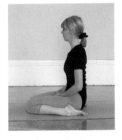

1 Kneel, spine straight, body facing forward. Bring thighs together, inner knee joints and ankle bones touching, tops of feet on floor, toes pointing back.

2 Put buttocks onto heels. Put palms onto the floor beside hips. Relax shoulders and arms.

3 Keeping knees together, take feet apart and with the hands, roll both calf muscles out to sides and down to floor. Put feet at outside of buttocks; toes point back, soles of feet face ceiling. Sit between feet.

4 Breathe in; stretch spine up, from tailbone to top of head. Open and expand front of the body, face looking straight ahead. Rest palms on front of thighs. (Relax arms and shoulders.)

5 Breathe out; keeping thighs together, roll front thigh muscles out to the sides. (Front of thighs face the ceiling, shins rest on the floor.)

6 Hold the posture and breathe normally. Stretch body upwards, keeping buttocks firmly on the floor.

Cobbler
(Baddha Konasana)

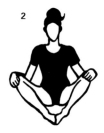

*shoulders low, relaxed
and parallel*

*front of body stretches
upwards*

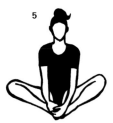

*spine and back of neck
lengthen*

*inner thigh and calf
muscles roll upwards
(to the ceiling)*

CAUTIONS

- Do not attempt if you have severe knee problems

- Never push the knees down with the hands

BENEFITS

- Strengthens leg muscles
- Stimulates abdominal organs
- Helps urinary-related, menstrual problems
- Relieves lower-back pain

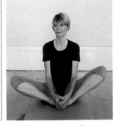

1 Sit in Rod or Staff (*p. 82*), basis of many seated poses.

2 Bend knees out to sides and bring soles of feet together in front of the body.

3 Clasp hands, interlinking fingers around toes of both feet; draw heels in towards crotch (outside edges of both feet and little toes remain on the floor).

4 Breathe in; stretch spine upwards from tailbone to top of head. Open and stretch up the front of the body, keeping shoulders relaxed and parallel.

5 Breathe out; push knees out to each side, rolling inner calf and thigh muscles up towards the ceiling (feel thighs easing out from hip joints).

6 Hold the posture, keeping spine straight and stretching the body up. On every out-breath, extend knees further out to each side; aim to bring outsides of legs and knees down onto the floor.

7 Take hands to outsides of knees, keep legs bent and bring them together, in towards body. Breathe out; stretch legs in front, relax arms by sides.

Easy Pose
(*Sukhasana*)
numbers correspond to instructions on p. 89

legs relaxed
arms relaxed
shoulders parallel
body extends upwards
spine straight

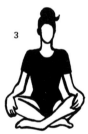

3

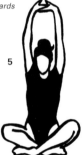

5

CAUTIONS

- Take care if you have a weak back
- Do not push the knees down to the floor

BENEFITS

- Strengthens the spine
- Encourages deep breathing
- Tones the nervous system
- Induces calmness in the body

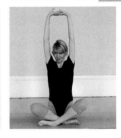

1 Sit in Rod or Staff (*p. 82*), basis of many seated poses.

2 Bend knees out to the sides.

3 Place top of right foot onto the floor in front of left shin; sole of right foot rolls up towards the ceiling. Place top of left foot onto the floor at inside of right thigh; sole of left foot rolls up towards the ceiling.

4 Bring knees in closer together, legs crossed in front of the body (tops of feet and buttocks stay on floor). Relax legs down to floor. Place palms on knees, fingers gently curved; relax arms and shoulders.

5 Breathe in; interlock fingers. Turn palms outwards as you raise your arms above head.

6 Hold the posture and breathe normally. Extend the body upwards on each in-breath.

7 Uncross legs and stretch them out in front; unclasp hands and relax arms by sides.

8 Repeat the posture to the other side, placing left foot in front of right shin.

Seated-Wide Leg Forward Bend

(Upavista Konasana)

numbers correspond to instructions on p. 91 and 93

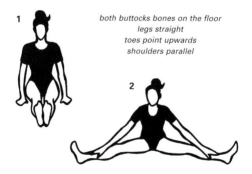

both buttocks bones on the floor
legs straight
toes point upwards
shoulders parallel

1

2

CAUTIONS

- Do not bounce into or in the posture
- Approach with care if you have back problems
- Take care if you have tight hamstring muscles

BENEFITS

- Stretches hamstrings
- Loosens hip joints
- Improves pelvic circulation
- Aids hernia problems

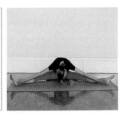

1 Sit in Rod or Staff (*p. 82*), basis of many seated poses.

2 Spread legs wide apart – 4 to 4.5 ft (legs should be the same distance apart from the body). Push heels away from the body; toes point up to the ceiling.

3 Keeping buttocks on the floor, hinge the body forward from hips and stretch arms down insides of the legs. Place the palms around the feet, or at any point that is comfortable on inside of the legs.

4 Breathe in; lift and open the front of the body, pulling abdomen muscles in and up. Stretch and lengthen spine from tailbone to top of head; pull in and concave the lower back.

5 Breathe out; extend and stretch the body forward from hips, leading with chest to flatten the back. Keep both buttocks on the floor, aiming to bring abdomen, chest and chin down onto the floor between legs.

continues on p. 93

Seated-Wide Leg Forward Bend

(continued)

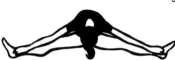

5 *shoulders parallel*
lower back area concave
both buttock bones on the floor

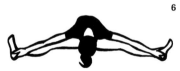

6 *legs straight*
toes point upwards

CAUTIONS

- Do not bounce into or in the posture
- Approach with care if you have back problems
- Take care if you have tight hamstring muscles

BENEFITS

- Helps gynaecological and menstrual problems

- Can relieve/release sciatic pain

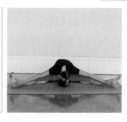

continued from p. 91

6 Breathe normally; on each out-breath extend and stretch the body further forward into the posture. Lengthen out spine and back of the neck. Relax head; push top of the head away from the body.

7 To come out: breathe in, raise the body to the vertical; breathe out, relax the arms by the sides, bring the legs together outstretched in front of the body.

Seated Forward Bend
(*Paschimottanasana*)

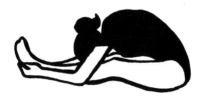

hands and arms relaxed
legs straight
toes point to the ceiling
whole of the back of the body stretches and extends

CAUTIONS

- Approach with care if you have back problems or sciatica
- Do not bounce in the posture

BENEFITS

- Excellent stretch to the whole back body
- Tones the kidneys and abdominal organs
- Improves digestion and circulation

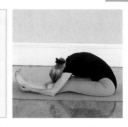

1 Sit in Rod or Staff (*p. 82*), basis of many seated poses.

2 Extend body forward, hingeing at hips; keep head up to flatten the back and bring hands down to feet. Place palms around outside of feet, or in any position that is comfortable on outside of the legs. Relax arms.

3 Push heels away from body, letting toes point to the ceiling.

4 Breathe in; stretch and lengthen spine from tailbone to top of head. Pull abdomen muscles in and up; open and extend body.

5 Breathe out; extend body forward, leading with chin. Aim to bring hips, abdomen and chest down onto front of thighs and put forehead on shins.

continues on p. 97

Seated Forward Bend
(continued)

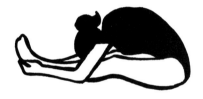

hands and arms relaxed
legs straight and knees locked out
toes point to the ceiling
whole of the back of the body stretches and extends

CAUTIONS

- Approach with care if you have back problems or sciatica

- Do not bounce in the posture

BENEFITS

- Induces calmness in the body
- Tones the kidneys and abdominal organs
- Improves digestion and circulation

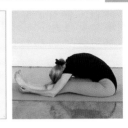

continued from p. 95

Push top of head away from body, lengthening spine and back of neck. Relax head and shoulders. Relax arms on the floor by sides.

6 Hold the posture – breathe normally – on each out-breath stretch and extend the body further forward, aiming to rest the whole of the front of the body down onto the legs. Keep the back flat.

7 Breathe in, raise the body and head to the vertical; breathe out, relax the arms by the sides, relax the legs.

Swan

(*Hamsasana*)

numbers correspond to instructions on p. 99

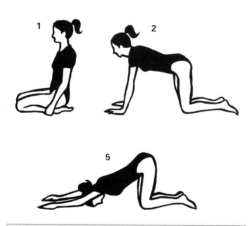

CAUTIONS

- Be careful if you have knee problems
- Approach with caution if you have back problems

BENEFITS

- Strengthens back and arm muscles
- Stretches the spine
- Tones buttock muscles
- Helps lower back pain

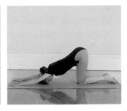

1 From kneeling position, come onto hands and knees.

2 Put hands, palms down, directly below shoulders; arms straight, fingers point forward.

3 Place knees directly below hips; shins and tops of feet rest on the floor, toes point back. Trunk is parallel to the floor.

4 Breathe in; raise head and look forward, open and expand front chest; pull in and concave lower back.

5 Breathe out; pulling in lower back, push tailbone back and up towards ceiling; simultaneously walk palms forward in front of body, shoulder-width apart. Straightening arms, extend and lower the body down towards floor; put head on the floor between arms (feel spine lengthen). Relax neck and head.

6 Hold the posture and breathe normally

7 Push buttocks back onto heels, allow arms and hands to slide back to sides. Breathe in; raise body and head to the vertical. Breathe out; relax arms by sides, stretch legs straight out in front.

Pose of a Child
(*Murha Januasana*)

whole of spine, back neck and head
lengthens (but is relaxed)

forehead rests on floor
or blanket/s

buttocks rest on
heels or blanket/s

toes point back

CAUTIONS

• Take care if you have knee problems

NOTES

• If the forehead does not extend down onto the
  floor, place a folded blanket/s in front of the
  knees and rest the forehead onto the blanket/s

• If the buttocks do not rest on the heels, place a
  folded blanket/s between the heels and the buttocks and rest the buttocks onto the blanket/s

BENEFITS

- Stretches the spine
- Eases tension in the back, legs
- Improves circulation to the head, face
- Encourages the whole body to relax

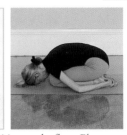

1 Come into a kneeling position on the floor. Place buttocks on heels, spine straight, body facing forward and arms relaxed by sides.

2 Bring legs together, inner ankle bones inner knee joints touching. Tops of the feet rest on the floor, toes point forward, front of thighs face the ceiling.

3 Breathe in; stretch spine upwards from tailbone to top of head. Open and expand front of the body.

4 Breathe out; extend the body forward, hinging at hips; lead with chin to flatten the back. Keep both buttocks on heels and place forehead on the floor in front of the knees (let front of the body rest on top of the thighs).

5 Place palms of the hands on soles of the feet. Relax back, neck and head.

6 Hold the posture and breathe normally.

It is important that the back of the body, spine, neck and head are relaxed in this posture; there should be no strain.

Corpse
(*Savasana*)

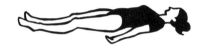

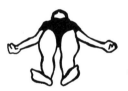

face relaxed, muscles soft
eyes closed softly
shoulders and hips parallel
arms and hands relaxed
front of body open
body in a straight line
back of body sinks into the floor
feet roll outwards to sides

NOTE

If the body is uncomfortable lying with the legs
outstretched, or if you have backache or back
problems, bend the knees up and place the soles
of the feet close in towards the buttocks, feet hip-
width apart, toes pointing forward. Relax the lower
back down onto the floor.

BENEFITS

- Relaxes whole body
- Releases muscle tension
- Calms nervous system
- Benefits heart problems

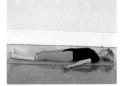

1 Lie, back flat on floor, body in a straight line, facing ceiling. Relax arms by sides, palms up. Close eyes.

2 Take feet hip-width apart; feet fall out to sides.

3 Relax lower back. Push shoulders down away from ears, stretch out back of neck.

4 Soften and relax facial muscles. Relax throat and front of neck. Swallow a few times; rest tongue loosely behind upper teeth; chin pointing to feet.

5 Relax pelvis, abdomen and diaphragm. Open and expand ribs and front of chest. Spread collar-bones out to sides (feel front of body open).

6 Relax the entire back of the body down into the floor, letting its weight be supported by the floor. The body is still and motionless.

7 Focus your attention on the breath; breathe through both nostrils and let your breathing slow down and become quiet. On each out-breath let the back of the body relax deeper into the floor; release and let go any physical, mental and emotional tension.

Sideways Hand-Big Toe

(*Anantasana*)

numbers correspond to instructions on p. 105 and 107

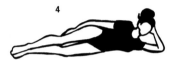

4

body weight
resting on
the left side

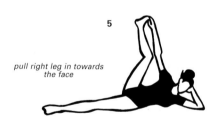

5

pull right leg in towards
the face

CAUTIONS

- Do not practise if you have arthritic hips
- Take care if you have problems or arthritis in the wrists or shoulders

BENEFITS

- Stretches hamstrings
- Stimulates leg muscles
- Helpful for back pain
- Increases hip mobility

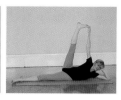

1 Lie with back flat on the floor, body in a straight line. Relax arms by sides; palms face the ceiling.

2 Turn and rest left side on the floor. Bring feet and legs together, with legs straight. Bend left arm at the elbow and place upper arm on the floor behind and beyond the head in line with the body; elbow points away from the body. Support head above the ear with palm of left hand.

3 Bring left side of the body into a straight line from elbow to heel. Push left armpit down into the floor (body weight resting on left side).

4 Put right arm and hand along the right side of the body.

5 Breathe in; bend right knee up towards face. Bring right arm and hand to the inside of right leg and hook the index finger and thumb of right hand around right big toe.

continues on p. 107

Sideways Hand-Big Toe
(*continued*)

*right leg and arm straight –
   extending upwards*

*left leg straight – heel pushing
   away from body*

*right side of body balanced
   directly above left side*

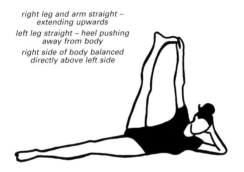

head and neck relaxed
straight line from left elbow to left heel

CAUTIONS

- Do not practise if you have arthritic hips
- Take care if you have problems or arthritis in the wrists or shoulders

BENEFITS

- Helps prevent hernia problems
- Tones pelvic area
- Stretches hamstrings

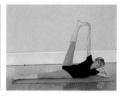

continues from p. 105

6 Breathe out; rotate right hip and leg up towards the ceiling (and holding right big toe with the index finger and thumb), stretch right leg and arm up to the vertical. Straighten right leg and push heel away from the body. Straighten right arm. Hold the posture and breathe normally.

7 Release the right big toe, bend the right knee down towards the face. Stretch the right leg out and place it on top of the left leg. Release the left arm from below the body. Turn and rest the back of the body on the floor. Relax the arms by the sides, palms face the ceiling.

8 Repeat on the right side from step 1.

Plank
(*Chaturanga Dandasana*)
numbers correspond to instructions on p. 109

1

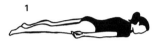

2

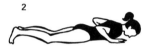

3

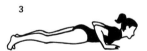

face looks straight ahead

shoulders parallel

upper arms strong

front chest opens and expands

legs straight

heels point forward

body in line with and parallel to the floor

CAUTIONS

- Do not practise if you have back problems

- Do not practise if you have arthritic wrists or shoulders

- Approach with care if you have arthritic hips or backache

BENEFITS

- Strengthens shoulders, arms, wrists
- Tones abdomen
- Strengthens leg muscles

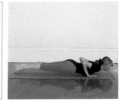

1 Lie with front flat on the floor, body in a straight line, legs together. Rest chin on the floor; face looks straight ahead. Relax arms by sides, palms to ceiling.

2 Take legs 12 in apart. Tuck toes under and push heels away from body. Pull kneecaps up and stretch out backs of legs.

3 Bend elbows and place palms on the floor at either side of the chest; fingers spread wide and point forward. Bring elbows close in, in line with shoulders.

4 Breathe in; raise chin and head; look straight ahead.

5 Breathe out; push body weight onto palms and toes and raise a few inches off the floor, keeping body parallel with the floor; face forward. Push shoulders up and back towards waist. Keeping toes on floor, push backs of legs up towards ceiling (feel the whole body strong, balancing its weight on palms and toes).

6 Hold the posture and breathe normally.

7 Breathe out; lower front onto the floor. Relax arms by sides, palms face up. Rest one side of head on the floor; relax the front of the body into the floor.

Fish

(*Matsyasana*)

numbers correspond to instructions on p. 111 and 113

2

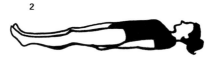

Most of the weight is borne by elbows and bottom

4

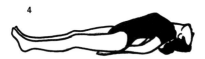

CAUTIONS

- Approach with caution if you have back problems
- Take care if you have neck or shoulder problems

BENEFITS

- Opens the chest
- Helps respiratory problems
- Eases neck tension

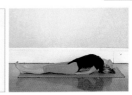

1 Lie with back flat on the floor, body in a straight line, legs together. Relax arms by the sides with palms facing the floor.

2 Slide right arm and hand under right side of body, and left arm and hand under left side. Palms rest on the floor below buttocks, fingers point towards feet.

3 Breathe in; raise head, shoulders, upper arms and body up off the floor (coming up to rest on forearms and palms). Keep buttocks and legs on the floor. Push front of the body forward and up towards the ceiling; open and expand the front chest.

4 Breathe out; push elbows down into the floor, curve the body back and lower top of head onto the floor. Arch back and raise front chest further up. Push heels away from the body, stretching.

5 For those who are more advanced: release arms and hands from below the body and bring hands into Namasti (prayer position) at front of the chest:

continues on p. 113

Fish
(*continued*)

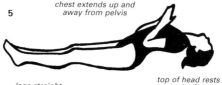

5

palms together – fingers
point to ceiling

chest extends up and
away from pelvis

legs straight

top of head rests
on the floor

relax shoulders – shoulders parallel
hips parallel

CAUTIONS

- Approach with caution if you have back problems
- Take care if you have neck or shoulder problems

BENEFITS

- Stimulates thyroid and para-thyroid glands
- Eases upper-body congestion
- Tones the heart

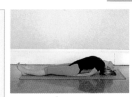

continued from p. 111

place heels of the hands at middle of the chest, fingers pointing up towards the ceiling.

6 Hold the posture, arching the back and breathe normally.

7 Bring arms down by the sides. Breathe out; push the palms down into the floor and slide the back of the head onto the floor, taking care not to stretch or strain the neck. Relax the back down onto the floor (lowering from the top to the bottom of the spine). Relax the arms by the sides, palms facing the ceiling. Relax the whole of the back of the body on the floor.

Locust
(Salabhasana)
numbers correspond to instructions on p. 115

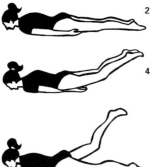

face looks forward

chin rests on the floor

arms and hands are relaxed below the body

spine extends, flexing back and up (at bottom)

pubic bone rests on the floor

legs together, stretching back and upwards

CAUTIONS

- Do not practise if you have abdominal problems
- Take care if you have back problems

NOTES

If you cannot raise both legs up off the floor behind the body, raise one at a time (*see 3rd figure above*).

BENEFITS

- Strengthens legs and lower-back muscles
- Firms buttock muscles
- Aids digestive problems
- Flexes spine

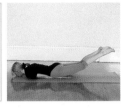

1 Lie, front on the floor, body in a straight line. Rest one side of head on the floor. Bring legs and feet together; tops of feet rest on the floor, toes point back. Relax arms by sides; palms face the ceiling.

2 Put chin on floor, face straight ahead. Slide right arm and hand under right side and left arm and hand under left side; palms rest at front of thighs, fingers point down to toes, arms rest on the floor.

3 Breathe in; keep chin on the floor. Push backs of arms and hands into the floor and raise both legs up behind the body, keep the pubic bone on the floor.

4 Breathe out; bring legs together and push toes away from body. Contract buttock muscles, push pubic bone and sacrum down to the floor and raise legs as high as possible off the floor.

5 Rest arms on the floor below the body, palms up.

6 Hold the posture, chin on floor; breathe normally.

7 Breathe out, lower legs to floor behind body. Relax arms by sides, palms facing ceiling. Rest head on one side on the floor.

Bow
(*Dhanurasana*)
numbers correspond to instructions on p. 117 and 119

1

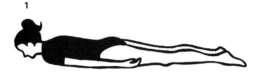

2

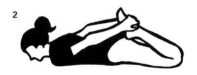

CAUTIONS

- Do not practise if you have abdominal problems
- Do not practise if you have high blood pressure
- Be careful if you have knee, hip or back problems

BENEFITS

- Expands the chest
- Brings flexibility to spine
- Beneficial for 'slipped disc' problems
- Relieves back pain
- Tones arms and legs
- Helps digestive problems

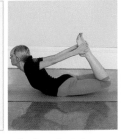

1 Lie with front of the body on the floor, body in a straight line. Rest one side of head on the floor. Bring legs and feet together; tops of feet rest on the floor, toes point back. Relax arms by sides.

2 Place chin on the floor. Bend knees and bring soles of feet up behind the body towards buttocks. Stretch arms and hands back, take hold of right ankle with the right hand, left ankle with left hand.

3 Breathe in; raise chin off the floor and look straight ahead.

4 Breathe out; push soles of feet up towards the ceiling away from the body. Pull ankles up with hands and raise knees and thighs up off the floor (both legs lift evenly). At the same time, raise the head, shoulders and chest off the floor, and come up to balance on the abdomen.

continues on p. 119

Bow
(*continued*)

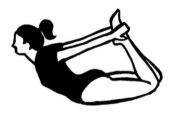

arms straight
the front of the body extends upwards
abdomen balances on the floor
soles of feet push upwards
lower back presses down towards the floor

CAUTIONS

- Do not practise if you have abdominal problems
- Do not practise if you have high blood pressure
- Be careful if you have knee, hip or back problems

BENEFITS

- Expands the chest
- Brings flexibility to spine
- Beneficial for 'slipped disc' problems
- Relieves back pain
- Tones arms and legs
- Helps digestive problems

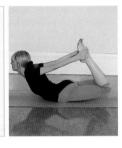

continues from p. 117

5 Bring the legs together with inner ankles, knees and thighs touching. Take shoulders back and push them down towards the floor, keeping them parallel. Slowly tilt head back.

6 Hold the posture, balancing on the abdomen and breathe normally.

7 Release the ankles. Breathe out; lower the knees to the floor and extend the legs straight out onto the floor behind the body. Push the palms down into the floor and lower the front of the body to the floor. Relax the arms by the sides; palms face the ceiling. Rest the head on one side. Relax the whole of the front of the body on the floor.

Cobra

(*Bhujangasana*)

numbers correspond to instructions on p. 121 and 123

2

4

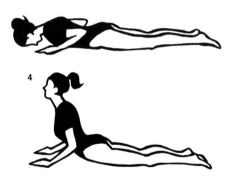

CAUTIONS

- Take care if you have back problems
- Do not practise if you have abdominal problems
- Take care if you have arthritic wrists or shoulders

BENEFITS

- Opens the chest
- Helps respiratory problems
- Strengthens pectorals
- Beneficial for 'slipped disc' problems

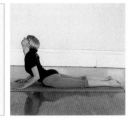

1 Lie with front of the body on the floor, body in a straight line. Rest one side of head on the floor. Bring legs and feet together; tops of feet rest on the floor, toes point back. Relax arms by sides, palms face the ceiling.

2 Place forehead on the floor and palms of hands directly below shoulders; fingers spread wide and point forward. Bring arms close to the sides of the body, arms bent with elbows pointing towards the feet.

3 Breathe in; raise head, shoulders and front of the body up off the floor (keeping pubic bone in contact with the floor).

4 Breathe out; push palms down into the floor and raise body up as high as possible (keep pubic bone on the floor). Open and expand the front of the body; face looks straight ahead.

continues on p. 123

Cobra
(*continued*)

5

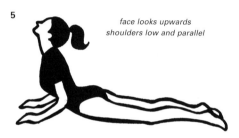

face looks upwards
shoulders low and parallel

front chest fully expands
spine extends; flexing back and up (at top)
pubic bone, coccyx and sacrum push down to the floor
buttocks relaxed
legs straight

CAUTIONS

- Take care if you have back problems
- Do not practise if you have abdominal problems
- Take care if you have arthritic wrists or shoulders

BENEFITS

- Strengthens pectorals
- Brings flexibility to spine
- Aids digestion
- Tones the buttocks

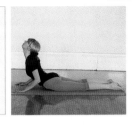

continues from p. 121

5 Take shoulders back; slowly drop head back and look uptowards the ceiling (arms may be bent).

6 Relax the buttocks and leg muscles (feel the spine extending and flexing back)

7 Hold the posture and breathe normally.

8 Push the palms into the floor. Breathe out; lower the front of the body down onto the floor. Rest one side of the head on the floor, relax the arms by the sides, palms face the ceiling. Relax the front of the body down into the floor.

Upward-Facing Dog
(*Urdha Mukha Svanasana*)

numbers correspond to instructions on p. 125 and 127

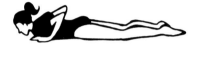

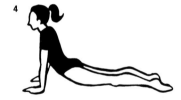

CAUTIONS

- Do not practise if you have severe abdominal problems

- Approach with care if you have eye, back or neck problems

- Do not drop the head back if you have stiffness or problems in the neck area

BENEFITS

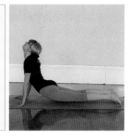

- Strengthens and flexes the spine
- Helps back ache/pain
- Beneficial for 'slipped disc' problems
- Opens front chest
- Tones pelvis, abdomen

1 Lie with front of the body on the floor, body in a straight line, legs together; tops of feet rest on the floor, toes point back. Rest one side of head on the floor. Relax arms by sides; palms of the hands face the ceiling.

2 Place chin on the floor. Take feet 12 in. apart, toes pointing back. Bend arms at elbows and place palms of hands on the floor at either side of the chest; fingers point forward. Bring arms close in beside the body; elbows point down to the floor.

3 Breathe in; push palms of hands and tops of feet into the floor. Raise up head, shoulders, body and legs a few inches off the floor.

4 Breathe out; straighten arms, pull body and legs forward, bringing the chest through in front of the arms (body curves back).

continues on p. 127

Upward-Facing Dog
(*continued*)

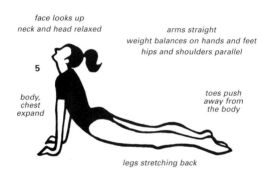

face looks up
neck and head relaxed

arms straight
weight balances on hands and feet
hips and shoulders parallel

5

body,
chest
expand

toes push
away from
the body

legs stretching back

CAUTIONS

- Do not practise if you have severe abdominal problems
- Approach with care if you have back or neck problems
- Do not drop the head back if you have stiffness or problems in the neck area

BENEFITS

- Strengthens and flexes the spine
- Helps back ache/pain
- Beneficial for 'slipped disc' problems
- Opens front chest
- Tones pelvis, abdomen

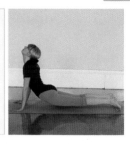

continues from p. 125

5 Roll shoulders back and push them down towards waist, keeping them parallel. Bring shoulder blades closer together; relax buttocks. Drop head back and look up (feel the front of the body open and expand).

6 Hold the posture, balancing body weight on palms and tops of feet, and breathe normally.

7 Breathe out; bend arms and lower the front of the legs and body to the floor. Relax head on one side, relax arms by the sides; palms face the ceiling.

Simple Twist
(*Bharadvajasana*)

numbers correspond to instructions on p. 129 and 131

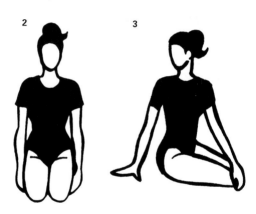

2

3

CAUTIONS

- Take care if you have back or knee problems
- Do not strain the back, neck or head

BENEFITS

- Strengthens and realigns the spine
- Eases backache
- Helps arthritis in spine
- Opens the chest
- Tones nervous system

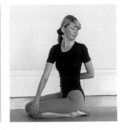

1 Sit in Rod or Staff (*p. 82*), basis of many of the seated poses.

2 Bend legs at knees and bring the lower legs back by the side of the left buttock; feet beside left buttock, knees point forward. Place right foot under left foot and rest hands, palms down, on the floor beside hips.

3 Place left hand, palm down, on the floor at the outside of right thigh. Slide left hand under right thigh; fingers point inward. Place right hand, palm down, onto the floor behind the body at base of spine.

4 Breathe in; extend and stretch the spine upwards from tailbone to top of head; open and expand the front of the body. Keep both buttocks on the floor.

5 Breathe out; rotate the body from the hips round to the right. Rotate the whole spine and bring left shoulder forward in line with right shoulder.

continues on p. 131

Simple Twist
(*continued*)

front and back views

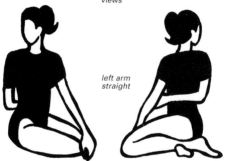

left arm straight

right angle at right arm
body stretches and extends upwards
body turns away from legs
legs together
knees point forward

CAUTIONS

- Take care if you have back or knee problems
- Do not strain the back, neck or head

BENEFITS

- Strengthens and realigns the spine
- Eases backache
- Helps arthritis in spine
- Opens the chest
- Tones nervous system

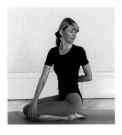

continues from p. 129

6 Keeping the left arm straight, take hold of the left upper arm with the right hand. Turn the head and look over the right shoulder.

7 Hold the posture, breathe normally. On each in breath, stretch the body upwards, lifting and opening the chest; on each out breath, rotate the body from the hips further round to the right, keeping the buttocks firmly on the floor.

8 Breathe in; rotate the body to the front, relax the arms by the sides. Breathe out; extend the legs straight out in front of the body.

9 Repeat posture to the other side.

Lying Twist
(*Jathara Parivatanasana*)

numbers correspond to instructions on p. 133 and 135

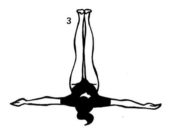

neck and head relaxed

arms straight – extending out from shoulder joints

legs straight (extend heels away from the body)

body and hips in line

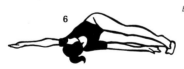

CAUTIONS

- Do not raise the legs straight, to the vertical, if you have abdominal or lower back problems

- Do not practise if you have arthritis in the hips

BENEFITS

- Strengthens intestines
- Reduces waist, hip flab
- Stimulates and tones abdominal organs

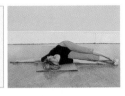

1 Lie flat on back, body in a straight line; shoulders and hips parallel. Relax arms by sides.

2 Extend arms out by sides at shoulder level; palms face the ceiling

3 Breathe in; raise both legs straight up to the vertical (can be done by bending knees over the stomach and then straightening them; see p. 134), push the heels towards the ceiling and flatten soles of feet; toes point in towards face.

4 Breathe out; rotate at right hip and slowly lower legs straight down towards the floor at right side of the body. If feet touch the floor, slide toes up towards right hand and push heels away from the body to stretch out backs of the legs.

5 Roll abdomen and stomach to the left and relax back of the body; keep left hip, ribcage and left shoulder down on the floor.

6 Keep both shoulders on the floor, shoulders parallel. Relax the neck and head and slowly turn the

continues on p. 135

Lying Twist
(*continued*)

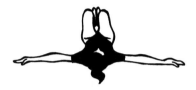

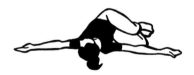

CAUTIONS

- Do not raise the legs straight, to the vertical, if you have abdominal or lower back problems

- Do not practise if you have arthritis in the hips

BENEFITS

- Helps gastric problems
- Eases lower-back, hip pain

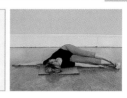

continues from p. 133

head to the left and look towards the left hand. Hold the posture, breathe normally

7 Push backs of the arms and hands into the floor and breathe in; raise the legs to the vertical and breathe out.

8 Repeat posture to the other side from step 3.

NOTES

If you cannot stretch both legs straight up to the vertical, bend the knees and bring them close to the chest, and take the legs down onto the floor at the sides of the body – with the legs bent (see illustration opposite).

Seated Spinal Twist
(*Maricyasana*)
numbers correspond to instructions on p. 137 and 139

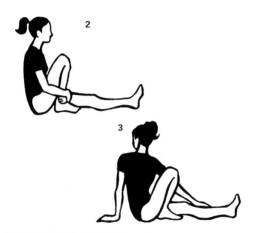

CAUTIONS

- Take care if you have abdominal problems
- Approach with care if you have backache or back problems

BENEFITS

- Opens the chest
- Relaxes tight shoulders
- Realigns the spine
- Beneficial for backache
- Tones abdomen
- Tones nervous system

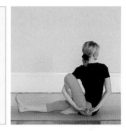

1 Sit in Rod or Staff (*p. 82*), basis of many seated poses.

2 Bend right leg and bring right heel close into right thigh; right knee points up to the ceiling. Extend left leg straight out in front of the body, push heel away from the body; toes point up to the ceiling

3 Stretch spine upwards and turn body from the hips, to the left. Take left arm back behind the body and place left palm down onto the floor at base of the spine, fingers pointing back and left arm straight.

4 Bring right arm to the inside of right leg and take it around the leg (from the inside to the outside) and bring the right hand behind the back. Raise left hand off the floor and clasp hands together behind the back.

5 Breathe in; extend and stretch spine upwards from tailbone to top of head; open and expand the front of the body.

continues on p. 139

Seated Spinal Twist
(*continued*)

4

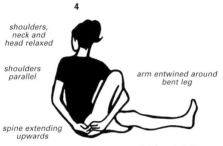

shoulders,
neck and
head relaxed

shoulders
parallel

arm entwined around
bent leg

spine extending
upwards

left leg straight
left toes point up to the ceiling

NOTES

If you cannot take hold of the hands behind the
back while keeping the spine straight: keep the left
palm down on the floor behind the body and place
the right arm at the inside of the right knee. Bend
the right arm, placing the elbow against the knee,
right forearm vertical with palm facing towards the
left leg; fingers point to the ceiling.

BENEFITS

- Opens the chest
- Relaxes tight shoulders
- Realigns the spine
- Beneficial for backache
- Tones abdomen
- Tones nervous system

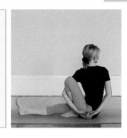

continues from p. 137

6 Breathe out; rotate body from the hips round to the left, rotating the whole of the spine. Keep the spine straight and bring right shoulder forward in line with left shoulder; turn head and look over left shoulder. Hold the posture – on each in-breath, extend and stretch the body upwards; on each out-breath, twist the body further round to the left, rotating at the hips; keep both buttocks on the floor.

7 Release the hands and relax the arms by the sides. Breathe in; rotate the body to the front, facing forward. Breathe out; extend the legs straight out in front of the body.

8 Repeat posture to the other side.

Boat
(*Ardha Navasana*)
numbers correspond to instructions on p. 141

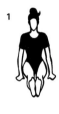

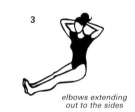

elbows extending out to the sides

legs straight

buttock bones in contact with the floor

toes in line with top of head

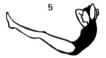

NOTES

- Do not let base of spine to come onto the floor
- Relax abdominal muscles
- If breathing is strained, breathe towards upper chest

BENEFITS

- Tones abdominal organs
- Strengthens back muscles
- Tones kidneys
- Helps trim waist

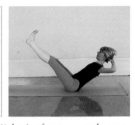

1 Sit in Rod or Staff (*p. 82*), basis of many seated poses.

2 Interlink fingers and place palms on base of head. Extend elbows out to the sides.

3 Breathe in; stretch spine upwards from tailbone to top of head. Open and stretch front of the body.

4 Breathe out; lean body back from base to a 30° angle and raise both legs straight out in front of the body to a 30° angle (buttock bones remain on the floor).

5 Push heels away from body, push back kneecaps and pull up with leg muscles and bones; point toes in to forehead (aim to bring toes in line with top of head).

6 Hold the posture, balanced, and breathe normally.

7 Breathe out; lower legs to floor in front of body. Straighten body to the vertical, release hands and relax arms and hands down by sides.

CAUTIONS

- Take care if you have abdominal or back problems
- Do not practise in the early stages of pregnancy

Boat With Oars
(*Paripurna Navasana*)

numbers correspond to instructions on p. 143

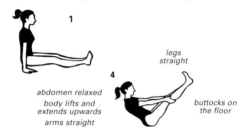

1

legs
straight

4

abdomen relaxed
body lifts and
extends upwards
arms straight

buttocks on
the floor

CAUTIONS

- Take care if you have abdominal or back problems
- Do not do if you have high blood pressure
- Do not practise in early stages of pregnancy

NOTES

- Keep lifting the body and opening the front chest
- Do not let base of spine come onto the floor
- Relax abdominal muscles
- If breathing is strained, breathe to upper chest

BENEFITS

- Aids 'bloated' abdomen, gastric problems
- Tones intestines, kidneys
- Strengthens back muscles
- Helps trim waistline

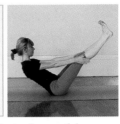

1 Sit in Rod or Staff (*p. 82*), basis of many of the seated poses.

2 Breathe in; stretch spine upwards from tailbone to top of head. Open and stretch up front of the body.

3 Breathe out; lean the body backwards from the base to a 60° degree angle and raise both legs straight up in front to a 60° degree angle. Toes point towards forehead, heels push away (feet are higher than the head). Buttock bones remain on the floor.

4 Extend arms straight out in front of the body keeping them in line with shoulders. Bring palms to the outside of the knees; palms face each other, fingers point forward.

5 Hold the posture, balancing on buttock bones, and breathe normally.

6 Breathe out; lower legs to the floor, straighten body to vertical and lower arms to sides.

Downward-Facing Dog
(*Adho Mukha Svanasana*)
numbers correspond to instructions on p. 145 and 147

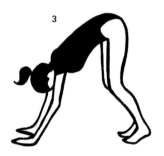

3

CAUTIONS

- Do not attempt if you have eye problems
- Take care if you have arthritic wrists
- Approach with care if you have high or low blood pressure

BENEFITS

- Stimulates the body
- Relieves tiredness
- Strengthens leg, arm joints, stretches spine

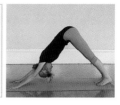

1 From kneeling, come up onto hands and knees.

2 Place hands, palms down, directly below shoulders, shoulder-width apart; fingers point forward. Place knees directly below the hips, hip-width apart. Tuck toes under; heels point up towards the ceiling.

3 Walk palms 6 in. forward (still shoulder-width apart). Keeping palms and toes on the floor, breathe out; push hips and tailbone up towards the ceiling. Push heels down towards the floor (feel the legs stretch out and strengthen).

4 Stretch arms out fully in front of the body, shoulder-width apart. Press heels of hands into the floor, squeeze shoulder blades together and push shoulders down towards waist.

5 Drop head and body down through the arms; top of the head faces the floor. Relax head and neck.

continues on p. 147

Downward-Facing Dog
(*continued*)

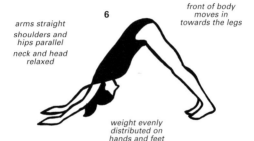

tailbone pushes up
towards the ceiling

front of body
moves in
towards the legs

6

arms straight
shoulders and
hips parallel
neck and head
relaxed

weight evenly
distributed on
hands and feet

CAUTIONS

- Take care if you have arthritic wrists
- Approach with care if you have high or low blood pressure
- Do not practise inverted postures if you have eye problems

BENEFITS

- Loosens hips, shoulders
- Increases circulation
- Stimulates the body
- Relieves tiredness

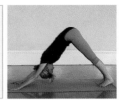

continues from p. 145

6 Push hands and heels down into the floor, push tail-bone up towards the ceiling and spread buttocks wide (the body's weight is evenly distributed between hands and feet). Hold the posture and breathe normally.

7 To come out: walk hands in towards feet. Bend knees and place them on the floor; shins and tops of feet rest on the floor, toes point back. Place the buttocks onto the heels, straighten the body up; body faces forward. Relax arms by sides.

Plough
(*Halasana*)
numbers correspond to instructions on p. 149 and 151

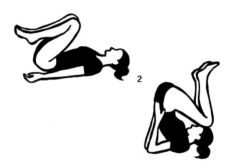

CAUTIONS

- Do not practise if you have high blood pressure, neck or shoulder problems
- Do not practise if you have lower back or hip problems
- Be careful if you practise this posture while menstruating

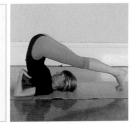

BENEFITS

- Stimulates thyroid gland
- Flexes spine
- Tones nervous system
- Stimulates abdominal organs

1 Lie flat on your back, body in a straight line. Relax arms the sides, palms on the floor.

2 Breathe in; bend knees up onto chest, push palms down into the floor and raise buttocks and hips off the floor to bring the knees towards the forehead. Place palms onto the back, supporting body, and straighten up the spine (bring elbows into line with shoulders).

3 Breathe out; extend legs out over past the face and bring toes down onto the floor; tuck toes under towards head.

4 Keeping toes on the floor, lift the ankles, shins, knees and thighs and push them up towards the ceiling. Push heels away from the body, straightening the legs.

continues on p. 151

Plough
(*continued*)

buttock bones push up towards the ceiling

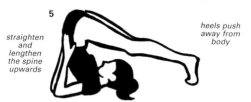

straighten and lengthen the spine upwards

heels push away from body

legs straight
front and sides of body open

NOTES

- If you cannot take the toes down onto the floor behind the head, place the toes onto a folded blanket/s or onto a chair.

- If you can take the posture further, bring the arms and hands down onto the floor in front of the body. Interlink the fingers and push the palms away from the body, with outside edges of the hands and little fingers resting on the floor. Straighten arms, lock out elbows and push the arms down into the floor. Stretch the spine up to the ceiling.

BENEFITS

- Aids digestive problems, high blood pressure
- Flexes spine
- Improves circulation, re-energises body

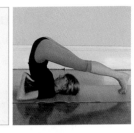

continues from p. 149

5 Bring palms up towards shoulder blades. Push the buttock bones up towards the ceiling, straightening and stretching the spine and spreading the buttocks wide.

6 Hold the posture and breathe normally

7 To come out: breathe out, bring the arms down onto the floor in front of the body, keeping them straight in line with the shoulders. Push palms and arms down into the floor and, keeping the back of the head on the floor, slowly uncurl the spine down onto the floor. Bring the legs to the vertical and lower them down in front of the body to the floor (legs can be bent). Relax back of the body to the floor, relax arms by the sides, legs outstretched in front of the body.

Bridge
(*Setu Bandha*)
numbers correspond to instructions on p. 153 and 155

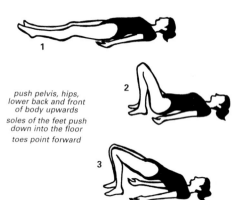

push pelvis, hips, lower back and front of body upwards

soles of the feet push down into the floor

toes point forward

CAUTIONS

- Do not practise if you have severe abdominal problems
- Do not practise if you have stiff or arthritic hips
- Be careful if you have back or knee problems

BENEFITS

- Opens front of body
- Helps respiratory problems
- Flexes spine
- Tones nervous system
- Strengthens legs
- Tones thighs, hips

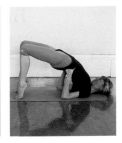

1 Lie, back flat on the floor, body in a straight line. Relax arms by sides, palms up.

2 Bend knees and place soles of feet flat on the floor. Bring heels close in towards buttocks, feet parallel, hip-width apart; toes point forward, knees point up towards the ceiling.

3 Breathe in; raise buttocks and back of the body up off the floor. Push soles of feet into the floor, tighten buttock and thigh muscles and push the pelvis, hips and front of the body up towards the ceiling. The body lifts upwards to rest on the shoulders.

4 Breathe out; place arms below the body, bend elbows and place palms of hands onto the back waist; upper arms stay in contact with the floor. Walk the heels (hip-width apart) closer in towards shoulders and push the pelvis, hips and front body

continues on p. 155

Bridge
(continued)

5

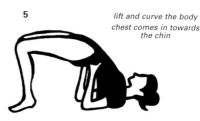

lift and curve the body
chest comes in towards
the chin

feet parallel
toes point forward

shoulders and back of head
rest on the floor

CAUTIONS

- Do not practise if you have severe abdominal problems
- Do not practise if you have stiff or arthritic hips
- Be careful if you have back or knee problems

BENEFITS

- Opens front of body
- Helps respiratory problems
- Flexes spine
- Tones nervous system
- Strengthens legs
- Tones thighs, hips

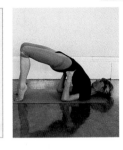

continues from p. 153

further up towards the ceiling, extending and pushing the knees forwards towards the feet (knees hip-width apart).

5 Relax shoulders and back of head on the floor. Tuck chin in towards chest to lengthen back of neck (feel the body lift upwards and curve back).

6 Hold the posture and breathe normally, balancing the body weight on soles of feet, shoulders and back of the head. (A variation is to come up on toes.)

7 Breathe out; bring arms down by sides, palms down. Push palms and arms into the floor and slowly uncurl the spine from top to bottom down onto the floor. Relax back on the floor, stretch legs straight out in front of the body and relax arms by sides.

Legs Up Wall
(*Viparita Karani*)

numbers correspond to instructions on p. 157

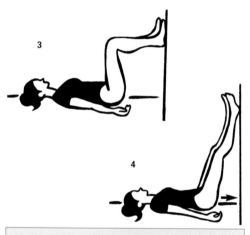

CAUTIONS

- Take care if you have arthritic hips/hip problems
- Do not take the arms over the head if you have a heart condition or high or low blood pressure

BENEFITS

- Improves lower-body circulation
- Rejuvenates tired legs
- Opens front of the body
- Releases lower-back tension
- Relaxes the whole body

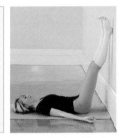

1 Lie, back on floor, with legs outstretched and heels resting on a wall. Relax arms by sides, palms up.

2 Bend knees to chest; bring buttocks in towards wall.

3 With knees bent, place soles of feet on wall, hip-width apart.

4 Bring buttocks in to touch the wall and extend legs straight up, together. Push heels up; toes point towards head (back rests on the floor).

5 Take arms over past head, arms slightly bent, and relax them onto the floor; palms face the ceiling.

6 Relax back of the body down onto the floor, ensuring hips and shoulders are parallel; legs rest in a vertical position up against the wall.

7 Hold the posture and breathe normally

8 Bring arms forward by the sides. Push the body back from the wall, bring legs down to the floor and straighten them. Relax the back.

RELAXATION

> *Lying full length on the back like a corpse is called savasana. With this asana tiredness caused by other asanas is eliminated; it also promotes calmness of mind.*
> Hatha Yoga Pradipika

Relaxation is an important element of yoga. Its purpose is to bring a stillness in the body and mind and eliminate outside thoughts, so letting you concentrate – the first step to meditation. The art of relaxation is also a very useful skill to learn: once mastered, it can be applied at other times – stuck in traffic, dealing with deadlines or coping with family rows.

BENEFITS OF RELAXATION

- Refreshes mind and body
- Invigorates nerve cells
- Increases creativity
- Promotes a calm and clear mind
- Lowers blood pressure
- Increases blood supply, bringing oxygen and nutrients to vital organs
- Can be practised in tense situations

A relaxation session should always come at the end of a class or your own personal yoga practice. Ideally, it should last for at least 10 minutes (but this also depends on the length of the yoga session; see p. 177).

PRACTICAL CONSIDERATIONS

The room should be at a comfortable temperature. The body cools down very quickly when lying still and if you begin to feel cool you will be unable to relax, so make sure you have a jumper and socks to put on or a blanket to cover yourself. If your neck feels strained, support it and your head with a small pillow or padding. Minimise distractions like TV, traffic or music. Half-draw the curtains to darken the room and make sure no-one will disturb you. Turn off the phone.

Basic Relaxation

1 Lie in Corpse (*see p. 102*).

2 Make sure your body is in line: head, chest, hips and ankles.

3 Feet should be a few inches apart, falling outwards.

4 Arms lie alongside the body, hands a few inches from the hips. Palms face the ceiling (this opens the chest) with your fingers gently curled.

5 Neck should be long with the chin slightly tucked in. If it doesn't feel long, lift your head up slightly, then lay it down vertebra by vertebra. Alternatively, place a small pillow beneath the nape of your neck.

Now that you are in the correct position, try to be aware of any tension points in your body.

<small>THINGS TO LOOK OUT FOR</small>

- Is your lower back tense? Is there a large gap between your lower back and the ground? As much as possible of your spine should touch the ground. Slip your hand under the small of your back then try to relax so your back sinks onto the back of your hand. Alternatively, place a cushion beneath your knees; this will help to lower your back.

- Are your shoulders creeping up to meet your ears? Shoulders should be wide and relaxed and your neck should be long. It is important not to let neck muscles contract and scrunch up. If you need to, place a small cushion beneath the nape of the neck.

- Is there tension in your face? Are your mouth and jaws clenched? Lips should be slightly parted, your tongue should even be relaxed. Eyes should be shut with the eyeballs soft beneath the relaxed lids. Feel as though you are smiling.

BREATHING

Breathing should be through the nostrils, slow,
steady, rhythmic. As you lie on the ground, become
aware of your breath. Don't force it, just observe
how it is coming and going. Watch how your tummy
rises and falls in a slow, regular rhythm.

HOW TO RELAX

Once you feel comfortable and relaxed, begin to release the tension from your body. Do this with each
part, starting with your feet and gradually moving up
to your head. Turn your attention to your:

1 feet – the skin on the soles, each one of your toes,
  insteps, ankles. *Feel them relax, grow soft and gentle.*

2 legs – calves, knees, thighs. *Feel them relax, grow
  soft and gentle and heavy.* Let the ground take the
  weight of your legs.

3 hips, buttocks and the muscles at the base of the
  spine. *Feel them relax, grow soft and gentle.*

4 waist, tummy, sides of the body, ribcage, top of the
  back. *Feel them relax, grow soft and gentle.*

5 shoulders; focus on the right shoulder and move
  down the right arm: top, elbow, forearm, wrist,
  palm of the hand, each finger in turn. *Feel them
  relax, grow soft and gentle.*

Focus on the left shoulder and move down the arm:

top, elbow, forearm, wrist, palm of the hand, each finger in turn. *Feel them relax, grow soft and gentle.*

6 neck, throat. *Feel them relax, grow soft and gentle.*

7 face – chin, lower jaw, mouth (let lips part slightly), tongue, cheeks, nose. *Feel them relax, grow soft and gentle.*

8 eyes – eyelids should be gently closed over the eye-balls, the eyeballs should be soft.

9 forehead, scalp, ears. There should be no frown lines. Your face is completely soft. *Feel them relax, grow soft and gentle.* Your head should be heavy on the floor. Your whole body should be fully relaxed.

As you become completely relaxed, you will feel the pull of gravity. Your body will feel heavier and heavier and you will let the ground take all the weight. You may not feel this the first time, but as you continue practising you will begin to recognise the feeling of total relaxation and it will be easier to achieve.

It is worth making a tape of the relaxation sequence for practising at home.

THE MIND DURING RELAXATION

At first it is hard not to let thoughts intrude. But tell yourself the relaxation session is a time to let your mind have a rest, too – it needs a chance to be completely blank. If you find thoughts flitting into your mind, push them gently aside, taking no notice of them. Gradually you feel divorced from your body as though you are floating outside it. It is as though you can observe yourself lying on the mat.

COMING OUT OF RELAXATION

When the relaxation session is over, it is time to take your awareness back to your body lying on the ground. If you are at a class, the teacher may have taken you on a visualisation journey to a beach or the country-side. Muscles and nerves have to be reawakened and brought back to the present. This is done by slowly moving fingers and toes, clenching and unclenching them. Then begin to stretch the body – hands and fingers stretch upwards along the ground, heels push downwards. As you stretch, let yourself yawn fully as though waking from a deep sleep. Stretch and yawn. To come up to a sitting position from Corpse, turn onto your right side and slowly push yourself up into a sitting position, taking care to let your head come up slowly. Keep your eyes looking down. Once up, slowly open your eyes.

YOGIC BREATHING

When the breath wanders (i.e. is irregular) the mind also is unsteady. But when the breath is calmed, the mind too will be still, and the yogi achieves long life. Therefore one should learn to control the breath.
Hatha Yoga Pradipika

Yogic breathing or *pranayama* is the fourth limb or stage of yoga (*see p. 184*) and comes after the postures or *asanas*. *Prana* has several meanings: breath, respiration, life, vitality, wind, energy and strength; while *yama* is restraint or discipline. The control of *prana* leads to the control of the mind which is vital for concentration and meditation, the next stages of yoga. But yogic breathing is also recognised as one of the main ways to refresh and rejuvenate all the body systems.

In yoga the breath is used to direct the flow of *prana* in the body. And just as blood circulates through a network of veins and arteries, *prana* is believed to flow through the body along a network of channels known as *nadi*. There are thought to be over 72,000 of these channels criss-crossing the body.

The main channel and most important nadi runs along the spinal column and is known as *sushumna*. For *prana* to move freely, it is essential there are no blockages. Just as a blocked pipe causes problems, a blockage of energy can cause havoc in the body and nervous system. Many of the yoga postures keep the spine flexible, thereby ensuring this main channel is clear.

Situated along the spine are centres of energy known as *chakras* (meaning wheel). There are believed to be seven of these and blockages can cause problems. For instance, a blockage in the Svadhisthana Chakra (in the genital area) can result in greed, lust or envy. A blockage in the Manipura Chakra (in the navel area) can result in anger and digestive disorders. A blockage in the Anahata Chakra, also known as the heart centre, might result in difficulty in expressing emotion. A blockage in the Vishuddha Chakra (in the throat) might result in a speech impediment, or thyroid problems. It is important to keep this main energy channel clear with the 'wheels' turning smoothly. So when you practise breathing it is essential to keep the spine erect. Some techniques can be practised lying down and you can even practise sitting on a chair, so long as your spine is straight. The illustration on the following page shows the seven chakras and their sites.

In this chapter we give the main yogic breathing techniques. It is always best to do these initially under the supervision of a qualified yoga teacher. If you are not taught these breathing exercises in class, don't be afraid to ask your teacher for advice and guidance.

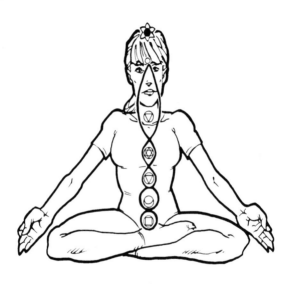

Symbols for each of the seven chakras are shown in their relative positions on the body

THE CHAKRAS

Sahasrara Chakra
location: crown of head
influences: pineal gland   *colour:* white/violet
represents: enlightenment, bliss   *mantra:* om (longer)

Anja Chakra
location: middle of forehead (third eye)
influences: pituitary gland,
         nervous system   *colour:* indigo
represents: intuition, wisdom   *mantra:* om (short)

Vishudda Chakra
location: throat
influences: thyroid gland, throat, lungs   *colour:* blue
represents: higher knowledge, learning   *mantra:* ham

Anahata Chakra
location: centre of chest (heart centre)
influences: heart and blood circulation   *colour:* green
represents: love, compassion, emotions *mantra:* yam

Manipura Chakra
location: navel (solar plexus)
influences: digestive system   *colour:* yellow
represents: will power, self assertion   *mantra:* ram

Svadhisthana Chakra
location: genital area
influences: reproduction, growth   *colour:* orange
represents: growth, preservation   *mantra:* vam

Muladhara Chakra
location: base of spine (anus)
influences: elimination processes   *colour:* red
represents: physical strength, stability   *mantra:* lam

BENEFITS OF YOGIC BREATHING
- Calms and quietens the mind
- Strengthens the immune system
- Improves concentration
- Increases the capacity of the lungs
- Refreshes both the body and mind
- Improves circulation of the blood

CAUTION

Pranayama is a powerful technique and care should be taken when practising. If you feel your breathing becoming uncomfortable or you feel dizzy, stop immediately, lie down and relax. If it makes you feel over-emotional you should stop.

WHEN AND WHERE TO PRACTISE

1 Try to practise regularly at the same time each day, preferably early in the morning or evening.
2 Practise in a clean, airy place, free from distractions.
3 Do not practise for at least two hours after a heavy meal.
4 Do not practise if you are hungry.
5 Empty your bladder and bowels before practising.

Complete Breath

Most people use only the top portion of their lungs to breathe. Full yogic breathing involves all the lungs – the top part beneath the collarbones and shoulders, the middle part beneath the

BENEFITS

- Teaches you how to breathe properly
- Improves quality of life

ribcage and the bottom part (the largest area) above the diaphragm.

Posture: seated or lying down

1 Pull in the abdomen and squeeze out the air from the bottom of the lungs. Relax the abdomen.

2 Inhale slowly and deeply, filling the bottom of the lungs (the tummy rises), the middle lungs (the sides of the ribcage expand) and upper lungs beneath the collar bone. Pause for a moment.

3 Exhale slowly and fully – first the top of the lungs should be emptied, then the middle area and finally the bottom of the lungs, pulling in the abdomen to make sure all the air is squeezed out. Pause for a moment.

Continue for as long as you like.

Cleansing Breath
(Ha breath)

Posture: seated or standing. Here, it is described in a standing position.

BENEFITS

- Empties lungs fully, expelling stale air
- Lowers carbon monoxide
- Benefits asthma and bronchitis sufferers

1 Stand with feet hip-width apart.

2 Inhale fully as you take your arms up sideways above your head.

3 Exhale through the mouth with a 'ha' sound as you bend forward at the waist. Arms swing through the legs; bend your knees slightly at the same time and pull in abdominal muscles to squeeze out all air from the bottom of the lungs; remain in the position without inhaling.

5 Exhale again through the mouth with a sigh to get rid of any further stale air in the lungs.

6 Inhale deeply as you straighten up with knees slightly bent. Arms come up sideways over your head.

Repeat three times.

CAUTIONS

- Do not do if you have high blood pressure, eye problems or a hiatus hernia
- Stop if you feel dizzy or hyperventilate

Alternate Nostril Breathing (Nadi Sodana)

Posture: seated

1 Sit comfortably with spine straight.

2 Take your right hand and fold the index and middle finger into your palm. The thumb, fourth and little fingers are straight (see right).

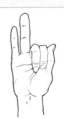

3 Close the right nostril with the thumb and inhale fully and slowly through the left nostril.

4 Close the left nostril with the fourth and little fingers and exhale through the right. Pause and then inhale through the same nostril (the right).

5 Close the right nostril and exhale through the left.

This completes one cycle. Start again inhaling through the left nostril. Only do three cycles to begin with.

> **BENEFITS**
> - Counteracts anxiety
> - Calms the mind
> - Promotes good sleep

> **CAUTION**
> - Avoid this if you have heart trouble

Victorious Breath
(Ujjayi breath)

*Posture: Easy Pose (p. 88)
or Hero (p. 84)*

> **BENEFITS**
> - Strengthens nervous system
> - Aids circulation
> - Improves lung tissue
> - Quietens the mind

1 Let your head fall forward onto your chest so your chin is pressed into your breastbone.

2 Stretch out your arms and rest the back of your hands on your knees. Join the tips of the index fingers and thumbs, leaving other fingers straight (this hand gesture is known as *hasta mudra*). Exhale fully.

3 Inhale slowly and steadily through the nostrils. As the air is drawn in there is a hissing sound (*sa*) caused by the chin lock. Fill the lungs and pause.

4 Exhale slowly and steadily. The air brushing past the palate will again make a sound (*ha*). Once the lungs are empty, pause.

Repeat for a few minutes with eyes closed. Focus on the two different sounds.

> **CAUTION**
> - Should not be practised by those with heart and lung problems

Bellows Breath
(Bhastrika)

Posture: seated

1 Inhale smoothly and deeply.
2 Exhale forcefully, using your abdominal muscles to push out the air through your nostrils. Feel as though you are trying to push something out of your nose.

BENEFITS
- Highly cleansing and invigorating
- Good for circulation
- Good for sinuses
- Clears mind and aids concentration

3 Relax your abdomen and air should automatically be sucked into your lungs.
4 Repeat the forced exhalation with the inhalation following. Picture a pair of bellows stoking a fire.

Practise initially for about 10 seconds. Once you master the technique you will be able to continue for longer. Stop immediately if you feel yourself becoming light-headed.

CAUTIONS
- Those suffering heart and lung trouble, or with abnormal blood pressure should avoid this
- Take care if you suffer eye and ear problems

Cooling Breath
(Sitali)

Posture: seated or lying down

1 Begin by breathing regularly.

2 Stick out your tongue and curl it into a tube.

3 Inhale slowly through the curled up tongue. You will feel the cold air on your tongue.

BENEFITS
- Relaxes nervous system
- Soothes eyes, ears
- Cooling
- Good for digestion and liver

4 Pull your tongue back in and close your mouth.

5 Exhale slowly through the nose.

Repeat as often as you like.

CAUTIONS
- Those suffering high blood pressure should avoid this
- Do not practise in very cold or hot air

Bee Breath
(Brahmari)

Posture: seated

1 Close your eyes. Lips and mouth should be relaxed.

2 Inhale slowly and deeply through the nostrils.

BENEFITS
- Helps insomnia
- Calms mind and soothes spirit
- Relaxes the body

3 As you breathe out slowly, make a humming sound like a bee. The sound should last for as long as the out breath.

4 Inhale slowly and deeply.

5 Exhale making the sound of the bee and focusing your mind on this sound.

You can practise the bee breath for as long as you like.

PRACTISING AT HOME

Success is not achieved '*by wearing yoga garments or by conversation about yoga, but only through tireless practice.*'
Hatha Yoga Pradipika

Ideally a yoga student will attend a class, perhaps weekly, and combine it with practice at home (although some students may not be able to get to a class and will have to learn from books or videos). However you learn, the key to success is perseverance in your practice. This does not mean setting aside an impossible amount of time – between ten and 15 minutes a day of personal practice is more realistic, manageable with a little effort, and far better than hour-long sporadic bouts perhaps once a week or so.

It is important to make yoga part of your daily routine so that if you happen to miss a session, you feel its absence and are keen to resume it the next day or week.

ESTABLISHING A ROUTINE

Yoga practice is generally done in the morning or evening, whichever is more practical for you. If you have to get children ready for school in the morning, an evening session is probably your best option.

HOW LONG SHOULD I PRACTISE FOR?

If you are a beginner, restrict your practice to ten minutes at first. Gradually increase this to 15 or 20 minutes as your stamina and strength increase. It is essential not to leave out the relaxation period at the end of a session. If you spend 15 minutes on practice, leave between three and five minutes for relaxation. Yoga should leave you feeling invigorated and refreshed, not tired. If you have the opportunity, you could also try a longer session, perhaps up to an hour, once a week.

WHERE SHOULD I PRACTISE?

Set aside somewhere to practise. It should be airy, clean and free from disturbance such as noise or interruption from other people. For example, it would be impossible to practise with a TV on. Make sure your practice place is uncluttered. You could dedicate this area to yoga by placing a picture there that you particularly like. If this image is always present when you practise, it will focus your mind on the yoga and help concentration. You could also have candles and oils. In the early stages you might find it useful to practise the postures in front of a mirror so that you can check that you are doing them correctly.

WHAT SHOULD I WEAR?

You should wear loose, comfortable clothing, with nothing on your feet. Try to keep what you wear just for your yoga practice; this will help focus your mind on what you are doing. White or cream-coloured clothing is ideal. Take off any jewellery that might distract you.

DO I NEED ANY EQUIPMENT?

Things which you might find useful are:

- a non-slip mat
- a blanket (such as a plaid)
- a chair (to use for some more difficult postures)
- a small cushion (to support the head or buttocks)
- a belt

WHAT SHOULD I DO BEFORE I START?

If you have decided to practise early in the morning, a hot shower or bath will get rid of any overnight stiffness. Brush your teeth and clear your nasal passages. Empty your bladder and bowels. Remember, you should not have a heavy meal before your yoga session. You can eat a light snack an hour beforehand.

Tell others in the house not to disturb you and take the phone off the hook or put on the answering machine.

GUIDELINES FOR YOUR PRACTICE

1 Move slowly and mindfully. Don't rush from posture to posture – hold each one for a few seconds.

2 Try to banish any outside thoughts; concentrate on the moment and what your body is doing – even the parts that aren't moving.

3 Go as far as feels comfortable. Remember, pain is nature's way of saying that you are going too far. The people who demonstrate postures in books are generally experts with many years' experience. You must not try to compete with them.

4 Breathe deeply and regularly; don't hold your breath.

5 Use the in-breath (inhalation) for lifting and opening into a posture and the out-breath (exhalation) to fold and relax into it.

WHAT SHOULD I DO IN MY PRACTICE?

Yoga is all about finding the correct balance. Balance should be reflected in the postures you choose; see the next page for a suggested programme.

You should begin a session with a few limbering up exercises, especially in the morning. These could include Cat (*p. 38*), Butterfly (*p. 36*) and the Pelvic Lift (*p. 40*). Alternatively you could do two or three rounds of Salute to the Sun (*p. 42*).

WHEN NOT TO PRACTISE

If you have a medical condition, consult your doctor before taking up yoga. You should also take advice from a qualified yoga teacher as to what postures you should avoid or modify.

Women who are menstruating should avoid inverted postures in the first few days. Pregnant women should seek the advice of a qualified yoga teacher on how to

SUGGESTED PRACTICE PROGRAMME

- **a pose that centres you**: Mountain (p. 48) or Tree (p. 50)

- **a side stretch**: Triangle (p. 52)

- **a forward bend**: Standing Forward Bend (p. 70) or Seated Forward Bend (p. 94)

- **a backbend**: Cobra (p. 120) or Upward-Facing Dog (p. 124)

- **an inverted pose**: Downward-Facing Dog (p. 144) or Plough (p. 148)

- **a twist**: such as Simple Twist (p. 128)

- **relaxation**: in Corpse (p. 102) for at least three or four minutes

adapt the postures. According to B K S Iyengar, all the postures can be practised in the first three months of pregnancy. You will be able to judge for yourself whether a posture feels right for you. Cobbler, which strengthens pelvic muscles, is a good pose for pregnant women. But the joints become much looser during pregnancy in preparation for the birth so it is important that you do not overdo any postures because you find you are suddenly more flexible than usual.

HOW TO STAY MOTIVATED

It is all too easy to start something with great enthusiasm, only to fall by the wayside after a few weeks. The secret to staying-power in yoga is discovering for yourself how much your life will benefit from it. Even if you later lapse for months or even years, one day you will find yourself coming back when the time is right or you find the right teacher.

These tips might help you avoid falling by the wayside:

- Find the right class for you and attend regularly. Make sure you leave work in plenty of time for an evening class and that you don't eat a big meal beforehand to give you an excuse not to attend.

- Make friends with people who attend your class.

- Try to attend a special day of yoga (often advertised in local yoga journals). A whole day spent devoted to yoga can be fulfilling and rekindle enthusiasm.

- Try out new postures in your daily routine and find out what effect they have on you.

- Get a friend interested and either practise together at home or attend the same class. The mutual encouragement is invaluable.

MORE ABOUT YOGA

> *When a man is attached neither to the sense-objects*
> *nor to works, and when he has renounced all desires*
> *of the heart, then he is said to have attained yoga.*
> Bhagavad Gita 6:4

We in the West practise yoga for a whole range of reasons, all of them perfectly legitimate. But its origins lie in Indian Hindu tradition. It is a physical, mental and spiritual technique which is believed to lead to liberation. To understand what is meant by liberation, you have to look at the meaning of the word 'yoga'. From the ancient Indian language Sanskrit, it means 'union' – the union between a human's individual consciousness and the Universal Consciousness. Some beliefs refer to this Universal Consciousness as God.

YOGA'S PLACE IN EVERYDAY LIFE

Yoga offers a means for humans to control their senses and cultivate a detachment from life, allowing them the freedom to go beyond the confines of their own experience. The yoga follower can gain freedom from the human condition and all that this might entail: sadness, happiness, illness, poverty, wealth and so on. This does not mean that you must lock yourself away from reality. Yoga is a philosophy rooted in everyday life and according to the classical yoga tradition there are four stages that a student must pass through:

Dharma Duty towards others and oneself; how you behave, and practise moderation in the way you live.

Artha Concerned with earning a living and being a householder – looking after yourself and family. This stage makes the student self-sufficient materially and teaches them love towards their family. It does not mean accumulating wealth, but letting yourself be comfortable so you can enjoy life.

Kama The enjoyment of life; only possible with a healthy body and balanced mind. This is where the yoga postures and breathing come in.

Moksha Freedom from worldly pleasures. This can be achieved through controlling the senses and looking inward by practising meditation.

TYPES OF YOGA

As explained in the first chapter, in the West yoga usually means hatha yoga. However, there are many different types, all leading to the same goal. Traditionally all these practices have been classified into four paths:

Jnana Yoga The path of knowledge or wisdom. It calls for self study and comes by meditation and detachment.

Bhakti Yoga The path of devotion and worship of the divine. In the Hindu religion there are thousands of gods and devotion to one or more of these is a way to yoga. This path is open to everyone – rich or poor, uneducated and educated. It just needs faith and love.

Karma Yoga The path of action achieved through selfless service to others. Two great examples of Karma yoga are Mahatma Gandhi and Mother Teresa.

Raja Yoga The yoga of mind and senses: the classical yoga. A branch of this is hatha yoga. Although yoga does not involve elaborate rituals, Raja yoga consists of an eight-fold path, or the eight limbs of yoga.

EIGHT-FOLD PATH

In the West many associate yoga purely with the physical aspect – the postures known as *asanas*. In fact, this is just one of the eight limbs. Imagine this eight-fold path as a very wide path to begin with which everyone can travel down. It gets progressively narrower with fewer and fewer people reaching the end.

1 **Yamas** Rules aimed at destroying our lower nature.

2 **Niyamas** Rules or disciplines aimed at improving our individual nature.

3 **Asanas** Postures aimed at controlling the body. Most Westerners think yoga is just the asanas and so are confused over what yoga is. By practising the asanas or postures one learns control over the body.

4 **Pranayama** Breath control; teaches one how to control the breath and direct prana, or life energy.

5 **Pratyahara** Withdrawal of the senses.

6 **Dharana** Concentration.

7 Dhyana Meditation.

8 Samadhi Union with the Universal Consciousness or God.

The first two limbs apply to everyone and consist of two sets of rules. The first are the *yamas* – rules people must follow if they are to live in a peaceful society. They ensure that no harm comes to any living creature either through thought, word or deed.

YAMAS

- non-violence
- truthfulness
- non-stealing
- continence or chastity
- non-greed

The other set is the five *niyamas*, concerned with improving the individual's own character.

NIYAMAS

- cleanliness (both of body and mind)
- contentment
- austerity
- self-study
- devotion to God or the Ultimate Truth

Once the individual incorporates these rules into his or her daily life, then they are ready to progress along the eight-fold path.

The next three limbs are *asanas, pranayama* and *pratyahara*. This withdrawal of the senses is where the student learns to distance him- or herself from external life and the distractions of the body and senses. Now the student will continue the quest for the ultimate truth by turning inwards. Some people might only get this far along the path.

The next two limbs of the eight-fold path are *dharma* (deep concentration) and *dhyana* (meditation). Once the follower has achieved this they may arrive at the final and eighth limb, *samadhi* or enlightenment where they are at one with the Universal Consciousness. It is not an easy path to follow: the individual must rise above the passions of everyday life (and actively want to do this) in order to get there. Ultimately there has to be complete understanding of his or her own nature. This in turn leads to the complete understanding of the Absolute or Universal truth of which we are all a part.

So yoga is not just a series of postures with odd names like cobra, locust and tree – it is a philosophy or way of life that is also very accessible. On the most basic level of the *yamas* and *niyamas* it shows humans how to live to ensure a peaceful society and one that will protect the world's resources for future generations.

Further Reading

If you want to read more on the subject, here are a few more suggested titles:

Light on Yoga B K S Iyengar, Thorsons 1991

Yoga Step by Step Cheryl Isaacson, Thorsons 1990

The Tree of Yoga B K S Iyengar, Thorsons 1994

Encyclopedic Dictionary of Yoga Georg Feuerstein, Unwin Hyman 1990

Yoga The Iyengar Way Silva, Mira & Shyam Mehta, Dorling Kindersley 1990

Yoga for Long Life Stella Weller, Thorsons 1997

Yoga for Women Paddy O'Brien, Thorsons 1991

The Ten-Point Way to Health Rajah of Aundh J M Dent & Sons Ltd 1971

Dynamic Yoga Godfrey Devereux, Thorsons 1998

YOGA TEXTS

Hatha Yoga Pradipika Yoga Swami Svatmarama, Thorsons 1992

The Bhagavad Gita Eknath Easwaran, Arkana 1988

The Upanishads Translated by Eknath Easwaran, Penguin Books 1988

Light on the Yoga Sutras of Patanjali B K S Iyengar, Thorsons 1993

Useful addresses

British Wheel of Yoga
1 Hamilton Place
Boston Road
Sleaford
Lincolnshire NG34 7ES
Tel 01529 306851

**Scottish Yoga Teachers'
Association**
26 Buckingham Terrace
Edinburgh EH4 3AE
Tel 0131 343 3553
Fax 07070 604380

Iyengar Yoga Institute
223a Randolph Avenue
London W9 1NL
Tel 020 7624 3080

Astanga or Power Yoga
Yoga Plus
177 Ditchling Road
Brighton BN1 6JB
Tel 01273 276175
E-mail
  yogaplus@pavilion.co.uk

Viniyoga Britian
105 Gales Drive
Three Bridges
Crawley RH10 1QD
Tel 01293 536664

**Sivananda Yoga Vedanta
Centre**
51 Felsham Road
London SW15 1AZ
Tel 020 8780 0160
E-mail
  siva@dial.pipex.com
http://www.sivananda.org

Kundalini Yoga
International Kundalini
Yoga Teachers' Association
Route 2, Box 4 Shady Lane
Espanola, NM 87532,
USA
Tel (001) 505 753 0423
Fax (001) 505 753 5982

Glossary of English/Sanskrit Names

ENGLISH	SANSKRIT
Boat	Ardha Navasana
Boat With Oars	Paripurna Navasana
Bow	Dhanurasana
Bridge	Setu Bandha
Cobbler	Baddha Konasana
Cobra	Bhujangasana
Corpse	Savasana
Downward-Facing Dog	Adho Mukha Svanasana
Easy Pose	Sukhasana
Fish	Matsyasana
Flank Stretch	Parsvakonasana
Half Moon	Ardha Chandrasana
Hero	Virasana
Legs Up Wall	Viparita Karani
Locust	Salabhasana
Lying Twist	Jathara Parivartanasana
Mountain	Tadasana
Plank	Chaturanga Dandasana
Plough	Halasana
Pose of a Child	Murha Janusasana
Rod	Dandasana
Salute to the Sun	Surya Namaskar
Seated Forward Bend	Paschimottanasana

Seated Spinal Twist	Maricyasana
Seated Wide-Leg Forward Bend	Upavista Konasana
Sideways Forward Bend	Parsvottanasana
Sideways Hand-Big Toe	Anantasana
Simple Twist	Bharadvajasana
Staff	Dandasana
Standing Forward Bend	Uttanasana
Swan	Hamsasana
Tree	Vrksasana
Triangle	Trikonasana
Upward-Facing dog	Urdhva Mukha Svanasana
Warrior I	Virabhadrasana I
Warrior II	Virabhadrasana II
Wide-leg Forward Bend	Prasarita Padottanasana

SANSKRIT	ENGLISH
Adho Mukha Svanasana	Downward-Facing Dog
Anantasana	Sideways Hand-Big Toe
Ardha Chandrasana	Half Moon
Ardha Navasana	Boat
Baddha Konasana	Cobbler
Bharadvajasana	Simple Twist
Bhujangasana	Cobra
Chaturanga Dandasana	Plank
Dandasana	Staff or Rod
Dhanurasana	Bow
Halasana	Plough
Hamsasana	Swan
Jathara Parivartanasana	Lying Twist
Maricyasana	Seated Spinal Twist
Matsyasana	Fish
Murha Janusasana	Pose of a Child
Paripurna Navasana	Boat With Oars
Parsvakonasana	Flank Stretch
Parsvottanasana	Sideways Forward Bend
Paschimottanasana	Seated Forward Bend
Prasarita Padottanasana	Wide-Leg Forward Bend
Salabhasana	Locust
Savasana	Corpse
Setu Bandha	Bridge
Sukhasana	Easy Pose
Surya Namaskar	Salute to the Sun
Tadasana	Mountain
Trikonasana	Triangle

Upavista Konasana	Seated Wide-Leg Forward Bend
Urdhva Mukha Svanasana	Upward-Facing Dog
Uttanasana	Standing Forward Bend
Viparita Karani	Legs Up Wall
Virabhadrasana I	Warrior I
Virabhadrasana II	Warrior II
Virasana	Hero
Vrksasana	Tree

COLLINS GEM
1950s
a mine of information

COLLINS GEM
1960s
a mine of information

COLLINS GEM
1970s
NO GAS
a mine of information

COLLINS GEM
1980s
a mine of information

COLLINS Jane's
CIVIL AIRCRAFT
a mine of information

COLLINS GEM
CLANS
& Tartans

COLLINS GEM
Classic
TV SERIES
a mine of information

COLLINS Jane's
COMBAT AIRCRAFT
a mine of information

COLLINS GEM
FIRSTS
a mine of information

COLLINS GEM
GOLF
a mine of information

COLLINS GEM
HILLWALKER'S
Survival Guide
a mine of information

COLLINS GEM
HOME
EMERGENCY GUIDE
a mine of information

COLLINS GEM
Collecting
STAMPS
a mine of information

COLLINS GEM
STARS
a mine of information

COLLINS GEM
SUPERSTITIONS
a mine of information

COLLINS GEM
Using Your
SOFTWARE
a mine of information